The Option of Parenthood

THE OPTION OF PARENTHOOD

Sue Dyson

sheldon**PRESS**

First published in Great Britain in 1993
Sheldon Press, SPCK, Marylebone Road, London NW1 4DU

© Sue Dyson 1993

All rights reserved. No part of this book may be reproduced or transmitted in any form or by any means, electronic or mechanical, including photocopying, recording, or by any information storage and retrieval system, without permission in writing from the publisher.

British Library Cataloguing in Publication Data
A catalogue record for this book is available from the British Library
ISBN 0-85969-649-9

Photoset by Deltatype Ltd, Ellesmere Port, Cheshire
Printed in Great Britain by Biddles Ltd, Guildford and King's Lynn

Contents

	Introduction	vii
1	Society's View of Parenthood	1
2	Why Do People Want Children?	13
3	Pause for Thought	28
4	Making Your Decision	57
5	Alternatives to Childbearing	70
6	Coping with Other People's Attitudes	88
7	The Rest of Your Life	96
	Further Reading	109
	Useful Addresses	110
	Index	115

Introduction

The choice of whether or not to start a family is essentially a modern one: only one or two generations ago, children were seen as the inevitable consequence of marriage. If you don't want children, as the saying ran, don't get married.

It is only with the advent of reliable contraception that parenthood has become the focus of heated debate. When childbirth was inevitable, there could be no question of a fulfilling, child-free relationship between a man and a woman. A married woman without children was the object of pity; sex meant children – its price or its reward. Parenthood can be deeply rewarding, but it can also be crippling. Is it for you? Infertility can be devastating but it can also be liberating. So is it really the end of the world? Is life without children really no life at all?

Nowadays, more and more people are approaching the prospect of parenthood with questions and mixed feelings. With the freedom of contraception comes choice, and choice brings anguish and doubt and the need for decisions. Society encourages parenthood, but not everyone wants – or is cut out – to be a parent. For some people the costs are too high – not just in medical, perhaps, or financial terms, but also in terms of strained relationships, thwarted ambition, loss of freedom, and environmental impact.

And the child? . . . surely parenthood is far too important a job to be allowed just to happen?

This book has been written to help you – and your partner – to thrash out the pros and cons of parenthood and what the reality would mean for you. It is also to encourage you to come to terms with how you really feel. There are no perfect decisions, absolutes, or guarantees. Only choice, and the responsibility of having made that choice. With honesty, insight and courage you can make – and take responsibility for – the choice that is right enough for you. Any choice brings loss, but it can also bring much personal growth, and a sense of fulfilment as an individual.

1
Society's View of Parenthood

In many people's minds, having children is 'the most natural thing to do in the world'. A woman's body has a built-in childbearing function, so is it natural that she should want to settle down and raise a family?

True, the *majority* of women *do* want to have babies, and *most* men say that they would like to become fathers. But that leaves a significant section of the population who either definitely don't want to have children, or who are undecided. Then there are the single people who might like to be parents, but have not yet found the right partner; lesbian and gay couples, and individuals wrestling with societal disapproval; and people who carry genetic disorders that may pose a risk to any future children they decide to have.

In short, parenthood is no longer the open-and-shut case it used to be. With the advent of reliable contraception, having children has changed from being an assumption, into a decision – a decision which is perhaps the most important that any individual or couple will ever make. Because of its importance, parenthood deserves to be thought about, discussed and debated at considerable length. And yet many commentators have remarked that most people give more consideration to the make of car they are going to buy than to the life-changing question of whether or not to have children.

Parenthood then, should be the result of a positive, informed choice, and not an unthinking reflex. And choosing is what this book is all about.

Unfortunately, the decision-making process is seldom allowed to operate in isolation. Individuals or couples thinking about having children are forced to negotiate a minefield of vested interests, media stereotypes, biased opinions and a host of other pressures. For society – even in this overcrowded age – still has its sights set on producing a nation of unquestioning parents.

Myths and motherhood

Since time immemorial, women have been encouraged to aspire to images of 'perfect' motherhood. In ancient times, when the world was young and life was hard, short and dangerous, it made sense to encourage women to produce as many offspring as they could. How else could the continuance of the race be assured? In such circumstances, it is hardly surprising that the very idea of motherhood should have become idealized. Nor is it surprising that women should have accepted the challenge, since for many centuries motherhood was the only way in which a woman could achieve success, fulfilment and praise.

Status was not easy for women to achieve in the Ancient World. In Greece, for example, women were seen as vastly inferior to men: a man who had lived a good and honourable life was said to return to his native star when he died; a less honourable man would be punished by being reincarnated as a woman. Even Aristotle concluded that women were no better than slaves. But the early Christians were scarcely more enlightened: St Paul was adamant that women must confine themselves to being subordinates, working to the glory of their husbands; St Augustine and Thomas Aquinas both asserted that woman's only function was as a breeder of children since in all other respects men were vastly superior.

Meanwhile, the cult of the Virgin Mary – which is, of course, still extremely powerful today – initiated the Christian tradition of idealizing motherhood. But Mary is a docile, submissive figure with none of the power of a matriarch. She is not a mother-goddess in her own right. She kneels before her son, acknowledging his superiority both as God and as man. Perhaps oddest of all is the fact that however hard women may strive to match this ideal of motherhood, they can never succeed, for Mary is what other mothers can never be: a virgin – and the mother of Christ. It is as though, whilst acknowledging the need for procreation, the Church is disparaging the way in which it is achieved.

Centuries later, Darwin's evolutionary theories served only to reinforce Victorian prejudices about women in general and mothers in particular. Women were considered 'less evolved' than their male counterparts, and in the thrall of their overwhelming biological urge to breed. Any woman who did not wish to have children, or who wished to fulfil herself in other ways, was considered unfeminine. The early 'blue-stockings' were condemned because it was thought that intellectual work would put too much strain on the women's minds and bodies, and render them barren. Even the sexologist Havelock Ellis believed that 'women's brains are . . . in their wombs'.

Faced with this overwhelming pressure, the near-impossibility of achieving economic independence, and the absence of effective contraception, women could do little but define themselves within the limits which had been placed upon them. Since motherhood was the only way in which they could achieve success and fulfilment, they determined to excel at it. They would be modest, strong, compassionate, unimpeachable, fertile and – above all – self-sacrificing, at every turn abandoning their own needs for those of their menfolk and their children. Inevitably, women themselves soon became the strongest advocates of 'perfect' motherhood.

Even today, we are not free of the man-made ideals of motherhood. The image of the Madonna and child haunts us still – the placid, contented mother cradling her baby son remains the epitome of fulfilment for many women. Ever conscious of the existence of our wombs, we have to make a conscious effort to be different – and even then, there is the gnawing doubt that perhaps we are making a mistake: that perhaps in being childless, we are cutting ourselves off from the ultimate mystery, the ultimate fulfilment of womankind.

In developing countries, motherhood is an essential condition of acceptance at all levels of society, and the only way in which a woman can prove her worth to the community. In Jamaica, for instance, a woman who has no children is referred to as a 'mule' – clearly signifying that she is seen as a working animal, and nothing more. The woman with many children is honoured and respected.

In many countries, the childless woman is described as being like a fallow field, or a tree which cannot bear fruit. If no children result from a marriage, it is assumed that the wife is at fault, and in some societies the wife is returned home to her father in disgrace, so that the husband can take another, more fertile, wife. No one stops to think that it might be the man who is infertile. The woman's primary task is to bear not her own children, or the children of the marriage, but her *husband's* children: she is, in other words, just the vessel in which they are carried.

Although some countries, such as India and Kenya, have

schemes designed to encourage a wider spacing between births through family planning and voluntary sterilization, it is still assumed that children will be born. And if a woman has a hysterectomy – for whatever reason – she risks losing her man.

In the West, just as in the developing world, mothers are still viewed as privileged, fulfilled beings whose lack of economic and political power is more than balanced by the influence, status and respect which they command at the very heart of the family. Women who are not mothers – however powerful their jobs may be – are incomplete and 'unfulfilled' creatures, full of regrets and bitterness. Small wonder then, that motherhood continues to appeal to the majority of women today.

Fatherhood and fertility

As we have seen, in a childless marriage it is rarely the man who is accused of being 'at fault'. Yet men who are in relationships may feel considerable pressure on them to 'prove themselves' by fathering one or more children.

Historically, whereas the mother of the child has been viewed as submissive, irrational, emotional and passive, the father has been portrayed as a strong stabilizing influence, the provider and protector. By acquiring children, a man could also acquire status and respect as a 'family man'.

Even in casual relationships, it is often not frowned upon for a man to father numerous children. AIDs is changing sexual behaviour slowly, but the onus is still often on the woman to take care of contraception. If a girl becomes pregnant, it is she who will suffer any stigma – plus the burden of deciding what to do about the pregnancy. The man may be on the receiving end of criticism, but he will also receive some tacit approval – he has 'proved his virility'. (And virility is routinely confused with fertility.)

The father may be required to contribute financially towards the upkeep of the child, but no man can be forced to take on the role of a father to his offspring. A woman can never forget a pregnancy, or a child to which she has given birth; but a man may father a child without even realizing it.

When governments play god

In Britain today, the official Government attitude towards

parenting is rather an equivocal one. On the one hand, there is constant pressure to conform to the ideal of the 'perfect' family, as a force for stability, a safety-net of community care for old and young, and as a means of instilling traditional moral values into young people. On the other hand, there is concern about overpopulation, unemployment and growing pressure on scarce resources in this tiny island.

Even with the introduction of social security benefits for single parents, life is difficult for a lone mother or father. It often seems that the message is that childbearing is generally a good thing, but only when the child is the product of a White, middle-class, two-parent, heterosexual family. The problem is that, even for those who *do* conform to these requirements, childbearing and rearing are no easy businesses: there are few financial incentives for women to have children, childcare provision is lamentable, and for most women, having children still means that their careers must suffer.

Similar conflicts exist in other Western countries, with the added complication that some governments openly admit to being worried about falling birth rates leading to an influx of immigrant workers. Some, as in France and Italy, pay premiums to women to encourage them to stay at home and have as many children as possible.

Back in Britain, the Welsh Nationalists have recently launched a campaign to encourage Welsh-speakers to:

> ... increase their families up to the limit they could afford – possibly four children – and rear their offspring in a wholly Welsh atmosphere.
>
> *Guardian*, 15 November 1990

Plaid Cymru has even suggested paying a cash bonus to the parents of a fifth child: a policy which has (not surprisingly) been compared to Nazi Germany's Mutterkreuz award for the mothers of more than four children.

Meanwhile, in some developing countries, governments struggle desperately to prevent their population growth from escalating to such a level as to spell inevitable famine and economic ruin for the country's inhabitants. India and China have well-known, if controversial, population control programmes; but even under China's rigidly controlled system, the population is continuing to grow at an alarming rate as couples defiantly assert what they believe is their moral right to have more than one child. Indeed, the United Nations Charter enshrines motherhood as a basic human right; and interestingly, the United States' Government recently offered political asylum to a Chinese woman who wished to give birth to more than one child.

A little further south, in Mexico, provincial authorities in the southern state of Chiapas have been forced to suspend the country's first-ever attempt at bringing in a relatively liberal abortion law, because of pressure from the Catholic Church. In many other countries – Britain included – a reduction in the resources available for family planning services is being coupled with attempts by pro-life groups to abolish or severely restrict the availability of legal abortion.

Doctors are joining in the debate, too – often contributing some very bizarre points of view. On 1 December 1989, *General Practitioner* magazine carried a letter from a family doctor, claiming that:

> ... successful, intelligent women [are choosing] to remain barren, depriving us of their offspring.

This is a viewpoint which has little basis in fact, since genetics do not work in quite such a simple way. There is no guarantee that the offspring of 'intelligent and successful' women will themselves be intelligent and successful; in fact, intelligence always tends towards the average.

Moreover, this outdated viewpoint has close links with the nineteenth-century argument against 'over-educating' women. If educated to a high standard, women might seek fulfilment in work or study, and would not marry, thus depriving society – and the Empire – of their childbearing potential. What's more, they would be so physically and mentally weakened by the unnatural effort of their studies that – if they did deign to marry – either they would be sterile or their children would be weak and sickly.

Individual governments, and influential bodies of opinion such as the medical profession, are quite prepared to manipulate their citizens either to encourage or suppress a desire to have children. Whether it is true or not, 45 per cent of Black South Africans believe that family planning is a plot by the government to reduce the Black population (according to the results of a DSI survey carried out in Johannesburg, Cape Town and Durban during 1990). And millions of Romanian women are still waiting to find out if their new government will carry out its threat to reinstate Ceauşescu's barbaric population policies.

In an ideal world, population planning and control would be viewed as a global issue, not as a competition to see who can breed the most 'racially pure' citizens and so influence the balance of world power. As it is, many developing nations feel that they are being asked to reduce their populations whilst the richer Western nations (who use most of the world's resources) expect to go on having as many children as they like. Population control is not a clear-cut, logical issue: it is tightly bound up with moral and ethical issues, and with individual desires and aspirations.

Ironically, in the countries of the West – where the extended family is almost extinct and the nuclear family disintegrating fast – it is the ideal of the two-parent, two-child family which governments are keenest to promote.

Yet Green considerations are certainly coming to the fore. More and more young people are looking at the evidence and making a positive choice whether or not to bring new lives into the world. As Joan Ruddock once remarked: 'We don't inherit this earth from our parents. We borrow it from our children'.

Media manipulations

In the so-called 'Caring Nineties', motherhood has become a watchword for all those 30-somethings who swore they would never have children but who are now approaching the menopause and wonder if they are going to miss out on what womanhood is all about. More and more women of 40 and over are deciding to have 'eleventh-hour' babies, and in Italy a 61 year-old obstetrician has given birth after lying about her age to get onto an *in vitro* fertilization (IVF) programme.

In the 1960s and 1970s, the emphasis of the Women's Movement was very much targeted on individual freedom. Women were busy asserting their freedom to do what they liked – to have careers, to have sexual relationships, to live as men lived, if that was what they wanted. There wasn't much room in all of this for children, as the feminist magazine *Spare Rib* noted back in 1987:

The issue became one of choosing, of what or who should be put first [job or home]. By deciding, as women, to put ourselves and our liberation first there was a feminist backlash against motherhood. The 'wife and mother' stereotype was forcefully rejected and child-bearing and -rearing became 'unfashionable' in many feminist circles.

In some ways this separated women from each other even further as those women who already had children or who wanted them felt that the women's movement 'disapproved'.

Spare Rib, January 1987

And then, in the 1970s and 1980s, along came the myth of the 'Superwoman': 'having it all' became the watchword of a generation of women who – to quote the women's magazine *She* – 'juggled their lives' between husband, family and career. Books, magazines, TV, films and shoulder pads ... they all built up a picture of the perfect wife, mother and career girl who could handle anything the world threw at her. Nobody stopped to ask if she should have to. The central truth – that every choice has a cost – became lost in the scramble to achieve the ultimate balancing act.

If anything, the 1990s have seen a shift away from feminism, and back towards a focus on parenthood as the ultimate fulfilment. So why the change of heart? It seems certain that media stereotypes have a lot to do with the sudden interest – among men as well as women – in becoming parents.

Advertisements bombard us with idealized images of parenthood: beautiful, fulfilled, successful parents with their happy, smiling, perfect offspring – no one is ever overweight, unattractive, bald, disabled, old ... and most of all, no one is ever unhappy. The message is clear: parenting will bring you happiness, fulfilment, a perfect lifestyle. If you do not have children, you are incomplete.

It isn't just women who are challenged by media propaganda. Men, too, are under pressure to become 'perfect' parents. It is no longer sufficient for a father to take on the odd stint of babysitting, under protest. The 'New Man' must follow a preconceptual health programme, support his partner unstintingly throughout pregnancy, be present at the birth, and get involved in just about every aspect of parenting – except breastfeeding. There are men who take to this new vocation like ducks to water, but others feel inadequate. And some mothers feel threatened, as though their partners are intruding on a uniquely female world. Most, if not all, fathers who try to become 'New Men' fail to match the media stereotypes.

So, for mothers and fathers alike, the legacy of media propaganda is dissatisfaction and a sense of guilt and failure. Media parents live in a world of contented, gurgling babies and perfect relationships. Real parents inhabit an altogether different planet – where exhausted parents yearn for a good night's sleep, where there is never a babysitter when you want one and where nappies always leak. 'Why isn't parenthood like it seems in the movies?' we wonder. I must be really bad at it. I must be a failure...

As *The Guardian* commented, on 30 January 1990:

> With bouncing babies and pregnant bellies pushed at us at every turn, those who choose to remain child-free can be made to feel distinctly out of step with the gurgling world around them.

Everybody's business

There can't be many people in the world who don't have something to say about parenthood. The question of childbearing is one on which everyone has an opinion – and unfortunately most people feel they have a right to express it in any way they like, even if it causes hurt or annoyance to others. Procreation isn't – and never has been – an entirely private matter between a man and a woman. Now, in fact, it's become everybody's business.

In this country, there is a tremendous division between parents and non-parents, and especially between mothers and non-mothers. Having children entitles you to membership of an exclusive club, to acceptance and approval by society. It isn't so much the number of children you have which brings approbation (in fact, society tends to look down on women who have large families): it's the very fact of being a parent. So having children becomes not just a matter of having them for their own sake, but having them to achieve status, acceptance and a link with the future of society.

The pressures from family, friends, parents, in-laws and society in general can be quite phenomenal. Garnette Bowler is a grandmother and retired health visitor, who has seen these pressures at work:

> The implication always is that you are not a fulfilled man or woman if you don't have children. . . . The majority do want to have children. But people are not abnormal because they think differently about responsible parenthood.
>
> The idea is supposed to be that having children is fun, natural and necessary. If you go against that you are saying it isn't all fun, it is hard work. It can be fun and joyous, but it can also be terrible. It can break marriages and it can destroy people.
>
> *Liverpool Daily Post*, 18 September 1990

Garnette is a very unusual grandmother. It is very easy for potential grandparents to forget that bringing up their family was hard work, and put pressure on their children to produce grandchildren. For, as grandparents, they can expect to enjoy all the fun aspects of bringing up children (days out, playing games, treats, presents, teaching and learning about the world), without any of the hassles and responsibilities. If a child is ill, grumpy or defiant, s/he only needs to be put up with until the end of the day, when s/he is delivered back to Mum and Dad.

Society looks favourably upon those who have children – though (as we shall see in Chapter 3) it makes only minimal efforts to provide facilities, support services and benefits for them. But society's attitude towards the childless or child-free is very different.

There are two stock responses to non-parents: pity and hostility. Initially, a childless woman or couple is likely to be regarded with pity, followed by incomprehension and even open hostility if it is revealed that the childlessness is voluntary. The hostility usually takes the form of an accusation that the childless person is being selfish. And yet, if parenthood is unfailingly and uniformly wonderful, why would anyone be foolish enough to deprive themselves of it?

The problem is so acute that many of the voluntarily childless let others believe that they are infertile – the pity is easier to deal with than the unpleasantness. For those who *do* have an infertility problem, and who have decided to opt for a positive, child-free life rather than an endless round of infertility treatments which may end in disappointment and failure, pity can be extremely hard to take. Yet it seems that society is not comfortable about encouraging positive, child-free living. In Chapter 2, we will look at the effects which these societal pressures have on individuals and couples who are deciding whether or not to have children.

Why society fears the childless

At the root of society's hostility towards the voluntarily childless is a deep-seated fear. If no one had children, the population would ultimately dwindle and die out. So society's interest is in persuading people to produce offspring, and it does so by creating images of parenthood as being not only desirable but the epitome of fun and fulfilment.

Voluntary childlessness is a direct challenge to this idealized image of parenthood. It brings into question all of the received values which society is at pains to instil. Fulfilled and happy childless individuals and couples pose a problem: if they are contented, how can parenthood be the only way to achieve fulfilment?

Men, too, may fear the woman who does not want children, claiming that she is 'unfeminine'. Even doctors sometimes join in the debate. Gordon Bourne FRSC FRCOG, author of the bestseller *Pregnancy* (Pan, 1975), claimed that natural selection determines childbearing. According to him, only the finest specimens of womanhood become mothers; less 'feminine' women become lesbians – an unconventional theory, to say the least.

As we have seen, traditional stereotypes of motherhood stress humility, selflessness, passivity. A woman who is not 'barefoot and pregnant' is far more difficult to control – particularly if she appears to be quite happy the way she is, deriving fulfilment from friends, career, and other areas of her life.

It seems that society's hostility towards the child-free is less about preventing society from dying out, than about making individuals – and particularly women – conform to an accepted stereotype. Society's 'ideal' woman is the Virgin Mary, not Lady Macbeth. Motherhood forces women into a nurturing role which keeps them out of the centre stage of politics and social agitation, makes them present themselves as soft and caring, rather than determined and strong. The family helps to control the male impulse, bringing male and female together in a union which protects the more vulnerable members of the unit. By contrast, child-free individuals and couples present a threat to the harmony of ordered social existence, since their ambitions and desires are not restricted by the need to protect and provide for their children. Small wonder that governments are so keen to idealize 'family values'.

2
Why Do People Want Children?

As we have seen, the whole of society is geared towards encouraging people to have children. Now let's examine some of these pressures in more detail, and see how they affect the decisions made by individuals and couples.

Social and family pressures: The price of belonging

Women are still defined in terms of their wombs, not only by society as a whole, but by their fellow women. Even today, when we have too many children rather than too few, parenthood is regarded as the desirable norm, for both men and women. According to conventional wisdom, a family is not a family until the children come along. This is particularly true in the case of women, for whom motherhood is an essential stage in their development, without which they cannot be admitted to the inner circle of female companionship.

There is always a tangible distance between the world of mothers and the world of non-mothers; and non-mothers who are not dedicated career-women tend to find themselves floundering in a no-man's land, unable to gain acceptance by either camp. Small surprise, then, that most women have children, since not to do so would go against the grain of everything around them.

Many childless women find that even the most long-standing friendships come under strain when their friends begin to have children. It is as though, if they want to retain their friendships, women must match the progression of each other's lives: school, work, marriage, children, part-time work, grandchildren ... Missing out on the all-important childbearing stage leaves a woman painfully out of step with her female friends. And men who are not fathers may also sense subtle changes in the patterns of their lives as, one by one, friends take up the challenges of fatherhood.

Of course, parents and non-parents can and do remain firm friends. But children are certainly a complicating factor, since they introduce parents to a whole new world of experience which non-parents cannot hope to share. Conversation becomes difficult, especially between a single career-woman and a full-time mother, since they have so few points of reference. The pressures are very much on the childless individual or couple to conform. All they need to do is have children, and they will be fully accepted once again.

On many occasions, childless (or child-free) women feel this pain of separation very keenly. There is so much pressure and propaganda, driving home the message that there is no happiness and no acceptance without motherhood. Childless women find that friends thrust their babies into their arms and expect them to respond immediately with a surge of 'maternal instinct'. Indeed, some women dread visiting their friends in the maternity ward, knowing that all eyes will be on them, and that they will be asked the inevitable question: 'When are you going to take the plunge?'

Many people – with no strong personal feelings for or against parenthood – end up having children not to please themselves, but to please other people. For example, one childless woman expresses her grief in terms of the need to satisfy other people's desires:

> My parents have no grandchildren, my dear husband has no baby of his own to love. I have this love in store to give to my child – love that cannot be used in any other way. I need to be loved and needed by my child, and I shall never be 'grown-up' as I shall never make the transition from being someone's child to being someone's parent.
>
> Newsletter of the *National Housewives' Register*, no. 38

Pressures – particularly from within the family – can be difficult to resist. Parents who want to be grandparents, and brothers and sisters who already have children, provide a ready-made frame of reference for a couple deciding whether or not to have their own children. Childless individuals and couples often feel that – intentionally or unintentionally – they are being squeezed out to the periphery of the family, no longer complete members with a full part to play in family events.

When all your closest friends are having babies, too, it can be difficult to resist the impulse to jump on the bandwagon. The fear of being left behind, or excluded, can be very acute.

On the other hand, it is all too easy to avoid making a positive decision, and blame any resulting problems on so-called 'external pressures'. As Renate Olins, Director of London Marriage Guidance, comments:

> There is real pressure, and there is imagined pressure. I think people sometimes say things as a way of denying that the pressure comes from within. They say, 'It's just my mother' – and that's not necessarily so. If we can blame somebody....

A survey carried out in 1991 by *New Woman* magazine and Boots the chemists suggested that external pressures are a good deal less important than many people claim. Sixty-one per cent of respondents said that they did not feel under any pressure to have children, and those who did feel pressure said that it came not from others, but from the march of time. Peak pressure seems to be felt in the early 30s, with 57 per cent of 30–34-year-olds feeling the most pressure at this time. This compares with 42 per cent of over-35s and only 8 per cent of 21–24-year-olds.

Those who felt under pressure from outside sources claimed that the most pressure came from their parents, and increased as they became older. However, few women claimed to feel under any pressure from their partners to have children.

It seems likely, as Renate Olins suggests, that external pressures can be magnified out of all proportion – particularly by a woman who is desperate to have a child. But where does that sense of desperation come from, if it is not from external factors? Scientific research has never satisfactorily proved the existence of a maternal instinct, though many women do undoubtedly experience a very strong urge to procreate. External pressures can provide useful excuses for people who want to have children, and who need to rationalize that desire to themselves. 'My mother keeps asking me when she's going to be a grandmother' sounds better than 'I want a child, but I'm not sure why'. Excuses like this help to remove the responsibility, too, if and when things go wrong: after all, you only had the child because your mother kept putting pressure on you, didn't you?!

According to child psychologist Dorothy Stein, there is no

doubt that parenthood – and motherhood in particular – has a lot to do with belonging:

> People can't disapprove of your having a child, so you can compel approval from other people. Most people say 'it's natural', or 'it's normal', blocking off an area they don't really want to think about too clearly.

Motherhood, fulfilment and control

Motherhood is one of today's most sought-after experiences; and yet it is not invariably a positive experience – whatever the media may wish us to think. Not all mothers fall hopelessly in love with their babies at first sight, and some never do. Recent statistics suggest that there are around 80 000 mothers in Britain living apart from their children, many of them voluntarily [Statistics taken from *Mummy doesn't live here any more – why women leave their children* by Helen Franks, Doubleday, 1990.] Clearly, there is a gulf in many cases between the image of parenthood and the experience of it, which begs the question: Why do so many women still desperately want to become mothers?

Much has been written about 'maternal instinct', and it is certainly true that many women feel desperately strong urges to bear children. A substantial proportion feel that, without motherhood, there can be no fulfilment. This view is summed up by Maggie Jones in her book *Trying to have a baby?* (Sheldon, 1984):

> (The woman) may desire the whole experience of pregnancy, birth, breastfeeding, motherhood – she may feel that she has not lived her life fully as a woman without these experiences. And then there is the simple, sensual joy of holding a new baby in your arms and providing it with the one thing it most needs and desires – love.

Or compare this view with that of Adrienne Rich, who writes in her book, *Of Woman Born*, of a meeting with a friend and her newborn baby. She recalls:

> a passionate longing to have, once again, such a small, new

being clasped against my body . . . how quickly one forgets the pure pleasure of having this new creature, immaculate, perfect.

In the twentieth century, motherhood has become an increasingly exclusive phenomenon. The relationship between mother and child has been idealized, deified almost. Mothers are expected to 'bond' with their offspring from the moment of birth, and to care for their children very much alone. Mother and child are supposed to become the focus of each other's lives, with no room for other women to share the joys and burdens of caring.

In this closed-off, hermetic world, it is hard for other women to share motherhood. If you want to find out what it is like to care for a child, you must give birth to one youself. We have grown suspicious of the old-world style of childcare in which many women share the care of the children, and the birth-mother is only one of the figures of love and strength with whom a child learns about the world. A childminder may spend time with the child, but she is a paid employee. Her relationship with the child ends with the termination of her contract. A child can have aunties and uncles and godparents, of course; but it can only have one mother.

Some lesbian women are particularly wary of getting too close to the children of their friends and lovers, since the tenuous relationship they have built up may be destroyed at any moment if the affair or friendship breaks down:

> I've never been happy about having relationships with women who have children. You see, you can get very attached to the children – but the minute the affair cools off, you lose touch. You're living on a knife-edge the whole time, hardly daring to get close to the kids in case you lose them. My sister's kids are different: they're my flesh and blood. As an auntie, I can enjoy sharing parenthood in a way I couldn't with a lover's children. There would always be an element of fear.

Perhaps it is these very fears which are persuading more and more lesbians, and other single women, to have their own birth-children. At least in this way, they will be creating a relationship which society will recognize, if not applaud.

No one has yet succeeded in establishing whether or not the urge to be a mother is inherent, or learned during childhood.

American sociobiologist Edward O. Wilson believed that the desire to give birth was 'programmed' into a woman's genes, but more recent opinion tends to give at least equal weight to the social and psychological pressures which women feel to reproduce.

Interestingly, surveys carried out by research psychologists have revealed that clinical depression is more common among mothers than among childless women – perhaps because the reality of motherhood so often fails to match the media dream, and because women are poorly prepared for the isolation and loss of status which new motherhood tends to bring with it.

But it is not the realities which most women consider when they make a decision to have a child. Very often, they don't articulate their reasons at all, and when they do they are often confused. In our world today, it seems that a simple desire to 'have a baby' – rather than a child – is sufficient justification.

Renate Olins, Director of London Marriage Guidance, feels that:

> some reasons for having children are better than others. One reason given is that if you don't have them, you might regret it later on – and I'm not sure that's good enough. The drive to have them needs to be more positive. I do feel that more people become parents than should do.
>
> One reason why people have children, and especially very young women, is to do with their own loneliness and sense of isolation. They want a little creature to love and who they think will love them. But to put that weight on a little human being is quite a worrying thing.

Child psychologist (and mother) Dorothy Stein is convinced that one of the fundamental driving-forces behind motherhood is the desire for control.

> I think, for women, the main motive is control. Women have problems controlling their own lives, and it has been found that women who have this problem often have children as an alternative. You find that legally and socially and in many other ways, children are considered as property, particularly of the mother (though formerly of the father). So mothers feel that they can choose and direct their children's lives to a greater

extent than their own: what they do, what they eat, what they wear, their names.

Also, women have children because they're a guarantee of unconditional, obligatory love. I've been on some television programmes, and what was interesting was that the people who were there defending childbearing got very upset with the people who had decided not to have children. They said, 'You are selfish', and they also said, 'I want someone to wipe the dribbles off my chin when I'm old'. They wanted someone to love them and keep them from being lonely when they were old.

She is also sceptical about the commonly held belief that the childless are either to be pitied, or cold and unfeeling people who despise children:

I have had experience with infertile people, and with people who have decided not to have children. And the idea that you have them because you like them is a myth, because the group of those who decided not to have them includes teachers, nurses, and others who work with children. On the other hand, the infertile seldom say they love children in general. But they often say they feel discriminated against or are considered defective.

The *New Woman*/Boots survey seems to confirm that many women, whilst wanting children, remain sketchy about their reasons for wanting to become mothers. Seventy-three per cent of respondents said that they had, quite simply, 'always wanted them'. Nearly one in five said that they thought having children would stengthen their relationship with their partners, and a further 20 per cent said that, having done everything else they wanted to do with their lives, they were now ready for a family. Interestingly, of those respondents who already had children, only 5 per cent felt that having children had strengthened their relationship. Twenty-eight per cent admitted that they couldn't explain why they had had children at all.

Tellingly, most women expressed their desire for motherhood not as a desire for children, but as a desire to 'have a baby'. It is relatively rare for would-be mothers to think beyond what Dorothy Stein calls the 'cuddly baby stage' to the months and years when babies become children and assert their existence as human beings. Indeed, some young parents actually ask their doctors, in all seriousness, at what age a baby 'becomes a human being'. Some women enjoy pregnancy, or adore small babies. Some see a child as a living doll which can be cuddled and dressed and controlled.

If there is a maternal instinct, an inherent genetic drive to reproduce, it seems that an increasing number of women either do not have it, or are choosing to deny it – without any obviously disastrous consequences. A significant and growing minority of women are deciding that they can achieve fulfilment only through *not* having children. Eighty per cent of respondents to the Boots survey said that they wanted children – leaving a substantial 20 per cent who didn't. This figure rose to nearly 50 per cent of all respondents over the age of 30. Perhaps more revealingly still, 12 per cent (and 39 per cent of over-35s) admitted that, if they were told that they could not have children, they would be relieved. Infertility would effectively 'let them off the hook'.

Nurse and Green campaigner Fiona Parkins lives with her partner Ted in a resolutely child-free relationship. She explains:

> I don't see parenthood as an unimportant job, it's just not for me. I can argue that I have lots more time – for other people's children, my friends or politics. It makes me more of a rounded person rather than feeling that I've missed out on my natural function.
>
> *Guardian*, 16 May 1990

Yet, as we saw in Chapter 1, society still finds it difficult to cope with women who do not allow themselves to be defined as mothers. Other women can be particularly hostile, as Carol Anne Davis relates:

> Get sterilised? You must be mad!
> You must first have a child or two.
> Don't want them? You're misguided, bad,
> Unnatural, of callous hue.
> *This be the verse: 1990 style*

Although more women than ever before are making lifelong careers for themselves, motherhood remains by far the easiest way in which a woman can define herself and gain the approval of those around her. Whether or not maternal instinct is a biological drive, it seems certain that social conditioning is an important element of the force which drives us to procreate.

As Sheila Kitzinger points out in her introduction to *In Search of Parenthood*, being defined in this way:

> shapes our self-perception and restricts our freedom to be other than wives and mothers. . . . The real denial of choice is not the inability to bear a child which is experienced by the infertile woman, but the social pressure on all women to have children in order to be able to ascribe meaning and purpose to our lives. The challenge confronting women is to claim our right to define who we are.
>
> <div align="right">Lasker and Borg, <i>In Search of Parenthood</i></div>

In Chapter 3, we shall be looking more closely at the process of choosing whether or not to become a mother, and at some of the factors which can complicate the decision.

Setting the seal on relationships

With the exception of single women who choose to achieve pregnancy through artificial insemination by an anonymous donor, all mothers have a relationship – however casual – with the father of their children. It is current Government policy to persuade fathers to accept greater responsibility for their children – even for children resulting from casual sexual encounters, and even when the mother would rather have nothing more to do with her partner. Yet, despite the current emphasis on parenthood as a joint venture, the decision to have children is often made by one parent alone. Frequently, it isn't even a conscious decision at all.

Many people see having a child as the ultimate expression of a loving relationship, the symbol of a perfect and enduring union. By having children, they are immortalizing their love and ensuring that their union leaves its mark on the world. Others view a child – unwisely – as a way of keeping a rocky relationship together. For some, having a child is a means of reliving their own happy childhood experiences, or of 'exorcizing' bad ones. In each of these cases, the child is being used as a means of satisfying parental desires, its own needs subsidiary to those of its parents.

On reflection, it is rather odd that society should see the childfree as 'selfish', since people tend to have children not for what they can offer the child, but for what the child can offer them (happiness, control, immortality or whatever).

> Jenni, a 16-year-old, had just left school and saw pregnancy (rather than motherhood) as a statement to the world about her relationship with the baby's father.
>
>> I'd been sleeping with my boyfriend for months, and it meant a lot to me. But he kept saying that just because we were sleeping together, it didn't mean anything. In the end, I decided to get pregnant so he wouldn't be able to deny that something important had been going on between us. I stopped taking the Pill, and got pregnant almost right away.
>
> She succeeded in making her statement but the relationship soon disintegrated, and she is facing life as a single parent.

Other women use pregnancy as an attempt to force their partner to make a long-term commitment. They feel – often wrongly – that once the baby arrives, their partner will grow to love it (and them) and will develop into the perfect husband and father. This rarely happens.

Having a baby to keep an unsteady relationship is also a risky business. More often than not, it has the opposite effect. Babies may be cuddly and loveable, but they can also be screaming bundles of tension and the innocent focus of both partners' accumulated acrimony. Where tensions and problems already exist, the arrival of a child will magnify them a thousand-fold in the first weeks and months of its life. What's more, it seems very unjust and irresponsible that an innocent child should be brought into the world, not for its own sake but as a sort of emotional 'cement' to heal its parents' rifts.

Paternity and potency

It isn't just women who want to have children. Most men also want to become parents. It seems that most men put forward two main reasons for wanting to become fathers: to pass on their genetic heritage to the next generation, and to prove their 'potency'. Less important seems to be the desire to have somebody or something to love – an important consideration for women contemplating motherhood – but once men have become fathers for the first time, this seems to become a factor in deciding whether or not to have more children.

It is quite odd that men should equate fatherhood with potency, since there is no link between a man's ability to perform sexually and his ability to father a child. A virtuoso lover may be completely sterile; whilst a man with a very low sex drive may have very active sperm. As someone once remarked, it doesn't deserve much praise simply to possess one spermatozoon with a sense of direction!

Nevertheless, the announcement of a wife or girlfriend's pregnancy is surrounded with congratulatory rituals for the father: the round of drinks in the pub, the cigars, the sly winks. Traditionally, male potency has been equated with power. In the days of high infant mortality and poor life expectancy, men wanted to have many strong, healthy sons who would look after them in their declining years and carry on the family line, inheriting their father's property and passing it on in turn to their sons. The laws of inheritance were firmly weighted in favour of male children until relatively recently, and of course succession to the British throne passes through the male line – princesses having no right of succession unless there are no male heirs.

There are still many men who admit to a strong preference for male children, or at least hope that the first child will be a son to carry on the family characteristics and name. Peer-group pressure can also be instrumental in persuading a man that he ought to become a father, if only to prove to his mates that he 'can do it'.

Research suggests that men are particularly keen that there should be a genetic connection between themselves and the children of the family: in other words, they are generally more reluctant than their womenfolk to consider options such as adoption and donor insemination. The reason for this may be that the father's only obvious contribution to the creation of a child is at the moment of conception, and this is, of course, a genetic contribution. The rest of the 'hard work' is done by the mother, over the next nine months or so, and her expanding girth is a natural focus for attention and approbation. If the father has no genetic link to the child which his partner brings into the family home, he may feel no link with it at all.

Dorothy Stein agrees that many men do have a positive desire to become parents, but adds:

> I'm not sure if they want them as much as women do. Most people don't think about it very much – they just assume that they will have them and enjoy 'family life'. I think if you asked them, some would say that they wanted sons, to carry on the 'name'. Perhaps they also feel that they can have with their sons a kind of relationship that they don't get elsewhere. Children are bound to look up to you, admire you, learn from you, love you. They are people you have a right to teach and discipline.

Just as some women submit to a partner's desire for a child, so some men give in to their partner's maternal urges – often thinking that, if they leave it all up to her, and don't get too involved in the practicalities of the child's upbringing, fatherhood may not have too much of an impact upon their lifestyle. Of course, the realities are rather different . . .

With the advent of the 'New Man' concept, more and more men are finding themselves expected to view parenting as a joint task. Whilst many men claim to take an active role in parenthood, most women still complain that their partners do not involve themselves sufficiently in household chores and in childcare. When they do, say the womenfolk, fathers tend to take on the 'fun' jobs like reading stories and playing games, whilst the mother is left with the chores, washing and dealing with toddlers' temper tantrums.

Nevertheless, there is evidence to suggest that – New Men or not – most fathers view having children as a positive experience in their lives. A research project carried out in America, back in 1960, asked 2 460 male interviewees what made them happiest – and relationships with their children came top of the list.

Opting out

As we have seen, having a child is not always a positive decision. Sometimes, it 'just happens'. And for some women, motherhood can seem a valid alternative to positive action, to competing, and to choosing.

Marina was 25 when she decided to have a baby. She admits that her decision had a lot to do with dissatisfaction with her own lifestyle:

> I'd had a succession of pretty boring office jobs since I left school, but when I was about 23 I decided to go off and do a training course to be a teacher. I finished the course, but afterwards I realized I didn't have the vocation I thought I had. I didn't want to be a teacher after all, and in any case there were hardly any jobs going. My husband was pretty keen to start a family, and to be honest I was fed up and quite fancied staying at home for a while. We could manage on one wage, but I didn't feel I could just stop working because I felt like it. But if I got pregnant, people would congratulate me and I could stop worrying about my useless career and where it was taking me.

Marina duly got pregnant and in due course had two children. She enjoyed looking after them while they were small, though she found the sudden isolation difficult to adjust to. It was when the children reached school age that the dissatisfaction started to creep back:

> I thought: 'That's it – I've done my job. They don't really need me any more. So what do I do now?' I realized I was going to have to stop trying to live my life through my children, and start making some hard decisions about what to do next. In the end, I found a part-time job and eased myself back that way. I'm glad I had the girls, but I can't help thinking that I had them for the wrong reasons. I'm only now beginning to try and achieve something for myself, and frankly I think I've left it a bit late.

For some women, the loss of autonomy which motherhood brings can seem like freedom: freedom from choosing, freedom from having to organize – and take real responsibility for – their own lives. What's more, it's an option which produces a generally favourable reaction from family and friends. But having children for such negative reasons can store up serious problems for the future.

The biological time-bomb

More and more women are having 'eleventh-hour' babies. It seems that some women do not feel the lack of children during their 20s and early 30s; but when they reach their mid-30s and the fear of increased risk of congenital abnormalities and even the menopause looms large on the horizon, they wonder if they ought to have a child now, before they 'miss the boat'.

It is at this make-or-break time that the woman is most vulnerable – to pressure from her own parents, for example. 'Are we going to be grandparents or not?' 'Are you going to let the family down?' Even a woman who has never felt in the least broody in the past is likely to experience feelings of panic as her options narrow: How many more fertile years have I left? Am I fertile at all? If I leave it any longer, will I increase the risk of having an abnormal child?

It can be hard for a woman to say a definite 'No' to motherhood when her biological clock is ticking away and soon the decision will be made for her. Harder still when she is surrounded by images of happy, fulfilled motherhood and cuddly, gurgling infants. Even a fulfilled career-woman can begin to wonder if having a baby might not make her life even better than it already is.

The fertility obsession

Most people don't give a thought to their fertility until they decide to start trying for a baby.

> Hilary and Hugh were in their mid-30s when a gynaecologist mentioned that Hilary might have problems in conceiving. Although Hilary had never classed herself as 'the maternal type', she panicked at the prospect of never being able to have a child at all. So she and Hugh decided to try for a baby straight away.
>
> At precisely that moment, Hilary was made redundant from a job which she really enjoyed. The redundancy came as quite a shock, and this was compounded when Hilary found that she had become pregnant, virtually straight away:
>
>> I couldn't believe it when I got pregnant straight away. Initially I felt slightly annoyed that I hadn't waited longer

after all. It's difficult to explain, but the speed with which it happened made it seem like an unplanned pregnancy – even though it wasn't. Maybe I just wasn't ready for it.

Hilary enjoyed her pregnancy, and was looking forward to becoming a mother. Yet when Toby was born, neither she nor Hugh felt any of the conventional feelings of warmth and affection towards the child. In fact, although they tried to conceal their feelings from each other and from other people, they resented the child and the changes which he had brought to their lives. Luckily, they were able to afford to employ a nanny; but even now, they have not really come to terms with parenthood. All in all, it is a tragedy both for the parents and for the child.

Cautionary tales like Hilary and Hugh's are a salutary reminder that parenthood is not always a joyful experience; and also that fears about fertility can propel people into making sudden and irrevocable choices which may not always be the right ones – for them or for the child.

Of course, infertility can bring untold misery to many people who have always longed for children; and there are plenty of people – men as well as women – willing to go to any lengths for even the slightest chance of parenthood. For these people, life is incomplete without a child, and no cost – emotional, physical or financial – is too great to pay in return for this chance. The quest for parenthood can quite easily become an obsession, and – like all obsessions – it can be almost impossible to view the issue in perspective and call a halt. Sometimes the obsession takes over to such a degree that the longed-for child is reduced to little more than a far-off, glittering prize.

3
Pause for Thought

Having children is a major, life-changing experience, so why is so little time and energy given to weighing up the issues and considering the responsibility involved? In this chapter, we are going to look at some situations in which becoming a parent raises specific, difficult questions.

The fertility issues

Fertility is one major medical factor that receives no attention at all until the moment something goes wrong. And at that moment, the discovery of infertility or subfertility problems brings about dramatic changes in relationships, self-esteem and perceptions of life, work and friends.

The vast majority of people take fertility for granted – until the day they decide to try for a baby. Yet infertility and sub-fertility are growing problems which affect thousands of couples in Britain every year. Around 80 per cent of couples will conceive normally after a year of unprotected intercourse – but that still leaves 20 per cent who will need help and advice. Some of these will never conceive at all.

The automatic reaction to fertility problems tends to be: what treatment can we get? Can we sign up for IVF or fertility drugs? Fertility treatments have progressed very significantly over the last couple of decades, and most couples can be helped. But fertility treatments require tremendous commitments in terms of time and flexibility – and sometimes money, too. The disappointment of year after year without a baby can destroy happy relationships and ruin a couple's financial security. At the end of the day, there may still be no baby. Some people are prepared to follow every possible course of treatment right through until there is nowhere left to turn. Others believe that there comes a time when they should call a halt. In many cases, it is easier to come to terms with childlessness if you have made a positive choice to stop treatment, since you retain a sense of control over your life and your fertility. If you are in this situation, you may find Chapter 4 of this book helps you to weigh up the issues.

According to the US National Center for Health Statistics, more than one in five American couples who want children have difficulty in conceiving or carrying a child: a total of over 12 million people, in one country alone. Other surveys have suggested that the number may be as high as one in three, and, for reasons which are not entirely clear, some experts feel that the problem of infertility is actually becoming more widespread. Even conservative estimates indicate that around one in six couples who try for a baby will have difficulty in producing a child.

Worries may lead to recriminations. Whose 'fault' is it? Although infertility still tends to be perceived as a female problem, the failure to produce a child is just as likely to be due to the male partner. The usual first step is to approach the GP, and from there on in the couple find themselves on a conveyor belt of treatment which it is quite difficult to get off. Examinations, investigations, sperm counts and postcoital tests lead on into the world of ovulation charts, bizarre sexual positions, loose underpants, high-protein diets; and if all else fails, to the high-tech hormone therapy, fertility drugs, surgery, gamete intrafallopian transfer (GIFT) and *in vitro* fertilization (IVF).

No one should underestimate the implications of becoming involved in a programme of infertility treatment. It isn't like taking a course of antibiotics, or just going along to the clinic every few weeks for a check-up. It's an all-consuming process that can easily take over your life and place considerable strain on your time, finances, health and personal relationships. This is particularly true if you opt for high-tech treatment and have to attend a private clinic, perhaps hundreds of miles from your home. Your normal daily life – job, home, friends, hobbies – everything ordinary and familiar is squeezed out by the all-consuming infertility programme, the quest for the ultimate goal.

And what if, at the end of the day, you do not achieve that goal? What if you find yourself without a baby, and also without friends, job, money, home? At what point should you say 'enough', and set about building a life without children?

Experts believe that some people continue with fertility treatments because they need an excuse – or rather *permission* – not to have children. They don't feel strong enough to tell the world that they don't particularly want children, so they go on with the treatments knowing that, if at the end of the programme they don't have a child, society will not blame them for not trying.

For others, fertility treatments become life's sole focus. Their desire to have a child becomes a rage, an anguish, an obsession. They feel discriminated against, because having a child is their *right*: they are being deprived of something which other people have no difficulty in achieving. Their pain is not only the grief of love unfulfilled, it is also the grief of failure and alienation. In extreme cases, the treatment may almost take the place of the desire for a child, destroying relationships, finances and harming the woman's health.

The costs – financial, emotional and practical – of *in vitro* fertilization (IVF) treatment are well documented. There are currently only two clinics in the UK which are funded entirely by the NHS, and these have enormous waiting lists. Some women are so desperate to conceive that they will do anything, pay anything. One woman – given 24 hours' notice to find £1000 for her treatment – was driven to 'borrow' the money from her employers, and ended up in court. Another spent a total of £19 000 over a period of ten years, and still ended up without a child. The average cost of IVF is around £1000 to £1500 per treatment, and the couple may have to undergo three or four treatments.

The psychological and emotional impact is no less grave. If you decide to embark on a programme of treatment, you will be placing all your hopes, all your dreams for the future, into the hands of a team of doctors. And at the end of the day, the success rate is not high. About 50 per cent of all women treated for infertility problems will conceive eventually, but only 10 per cent of those who undergo IVF treatment will eventually give birth to a live baby. In 1988, more than 7 500 women tried IVF. This resulted in 1 354 pregnancies but only 956 live births. Of the 43 licensed IVF clinics, two showed a success rate of less than 1 per cent over three years. Sadly, there are clinics and doctors who have no qualms about taking money from distraught women who they are virtually certain will never conceive.

The following letter appeared in the Autumn 1991 edition of *Issue*, a magazine published by the National Fertility Association (formerly the National Association of Childless Couples). I think it is worth printing here in full, as it gives such a vivid picture not only of the tragedy of infertility, but also of the agony and obsession which the prolonged quest for a baby can produce:

Dear Editor

I wonder how many other readers will identify with the day I have just had – and seem to have every day!

I woke up and was determined to take my husband's advice to 'just exist' through the day and not think too much (my downfall). Today, everything was just going to wash over me.

Sitting at work, those black thoughts started creeping in. 'BACK, BACK!', I cried, but to no avail. I am the only member of my family who is childless. My best friend, my sister, my sister-in-law and countless others have had babies this year, and my cousin is 6 months pregnant. I lost my second pregnancy this year through miscarriage (as well as my first pregnancy 18 months ago). It takes me years and fertility drugs to conceive, and so far an empty cot. Countless consultations and four operations have made no difference at the end of the day. It is truly a difficult time for me at the moment.

I try to put these thoughts far to the back of my mind and I go to do some photocopying. A young lad is staring at my red face (hot flushes are one of the side-effects of the drugs I am on) and I wish the floor would open and swallow him or me up!

I must try to be strong for my husband's sake, if not mine, I tell myself. A pregnant colleague is showing off her scan picture. I fight back my emotions.

Lunchtime, as I walk past Mothercare towards Boots, I pass loads of mothers and pregnant women, some posh, lots smiling, some clearly just out of school and I fight the urge to shout at them, 'Do you know how lucky you are?' But it's just going to all wash over me today; I must try really hard.

In Boots, lucky old me ends up queueing behind a heavily pregnant lady and has to endure the sales assistant's 'When is it due?'-type talk. All I wanted to do was to pay for my ovulation prediction kit, so my husband and I can try to put some variety into our baby making. I can't remember the last time we actually 'made love', it was years ago I know that.

That afternoon, I follow the mums around Safeways and my good intentions for the day are beginning to sag. On the way home I pass numerous cars with baby seats in and those hateful reminders: BABY ON BOARD stickers! There is no escape.

Feeling slightly safer back home, away from the real outside world I sit down with a cup of tea to read my magazine. Articles about babies, babies' clothes, babies' foods, the latest in maternity wear. Now I can feel the tension in me running from my headache right down my back and shoulders. Never mind, stiff upper lip and all that.

By the time my husband is home from work, he knows better than to ask me if I've had a good day. Over dinner I am quietly simmering on the verge of a total breakdown. We sit down to the delights of TV commercials for babies' foods and nappies and TV programmes where everyone apart from Eddie (who's just been bumped off in 'Eastenders') is pregnant.

I retire to bed exhausted. I feel a total failure for not being able to carry out my objective of letting nothing get to me. Anybody who thinks we can put it out of our minds and get on with our lives has obviously never been through it. Everything I do, everything I see, everywhere in my life there are reminders of my childlessness. It's so absurd, it's almost laughable! But I can assure you that I've had enough! So many years have been like this, sprinkled along the way with dashed hopes, desperation, tragic losses, depressions and illness and THERE IS NO ESCAPE.

I wish I could run away but there is nowhere to go where it wouldn't still be there. After all, you cannot escape from yourself.

I'm living in a society overrun with babies and motherhood, and I don't fit in. Yet I cannot give up wanting to become a mum. Broodiness doesn't go away – it just gets stronger. I will keep trying, therefore I must endure.

It is a sad letter, which shows how the desire for parenthood – and motherhood in particular – can squeeze everything else out of life. Friends, work, marriage, lovemaking – all are sacrificed on the altar of the quest. Couples may spend more than a decade of their lives simply trying for a baby, and putting the rest of their lives 'on hold'. But they cannot let go, because the next time, it might work. With the next ovulation, the next cycle of IVF, they may become parents! How can they give up until every last penny is exhausted, every ounce of effort expended? Whilst hope remains, grief can never be resolved. Until you call a halt, how can you come to terms with the rest of your life?

It is essential to weigh up the pros and cons before embarking on infertility treatment, and yet the medical profession does not always act responsibly. Couples have a need and a right to be told when the emotional and practical costs of treatment simply outweigh the likely chances of success. Otherwise, they will end up heartbroken and embittered.

MP Ann Widdecombe is critical of the tendency to view motherhood as a right, and suspects selfish motives in those who pursue treatments to the bitter end:

> The first question you must ask is, does a woman have a right to a child? Is it a right or a blessing? I believe that you should have a child for the child's sake rather than your own.
>
> The more I hear the long-term infertile talking, the more I realise they are obsessed with themselves and nearly always put it in terms of 'my needs'. A lot of what we see in the treatment of infertility is the exploitation of desire. I think it's reasonable that couples should receive treatment, but they should not be allowed to become so obsessed that they go on for ten years, possibly at the expense of others.
>
> 'Who has the right to have a baby?' *She* magazine April 1992

SCREENING

One solution to this distressing problem has been suggested by John Dickinson, Director of ISSUE. He believes that premarital fertility screening of couples who desperately want children could spare an awful lot of heartache later on. He explains:

> In recent times, the only person we know who was screened for fertility was Lady Diana, as she was then. It's simple to do, but everyone is so busy avoiding getting pregnant that they never think it would be a good idea to check their fertility.
>
> 'Who has the right to have a baby?' *She* magazine April 1992

No doubt the whole idea of fertility screening would prove repugnant to many couples, and destructive of the mystery and romance of courtship. But screening could prove to be the sensible answer for couples and individuals for whom having children is a major goal in life. Screening is easy to do, and is particularly useful in indicating to a woman how many fertile years she is likely to have in which to complete her family. At least by having herself screened, a woman can ensure that she doesn't leave it too late before trying to conceive.

ASSESSING THE REALITY OF YOUR CIRCUMSTANCES

In general, fertility decreases with age, and few doctors would be prepared to offer infertility treatments to a woman over 40.

Male sub-fertility can in some cases be treated, and donor insemination may be an option if you and your partner can come to terms with the psychological impact of having a child which is not genetically linked to both of you.

Around 50 per cent of couples who receive treatment will eventually conceive and produce a child. A significant proportion of these are helped by low-tech, low-cost treatments and natural techniques. For IVF, the success rate can be as low as 1 or 2 per cent, and conception is unlikely after three unsuccessful IVF cycles. There is also the cost to consider: it can often run into several thousand pounds, and of course, the disruption to your own and your partner's life.

If you try for a child, and discover that you have problems in conceiving, at the end of the day the decision must be yours – though you should ask your doctor for a candid explanation of what is on offer, and the likely chances of success. You have to take into consideration the whole range of personal factors, and decide whether you are prepared to put yourself – and your partner – through the rigours of treatment, bearing in mind that success rates are often disappointing. No doctor can promise you a child, no matter how desperately you want one. So are you prepared to sacrifice everything else that you value in your life, for a dream which may never come true?

Questions for you and your partner:

- How old am I?
- How old is my partner?
- Has a specific medical problem been identified?
- What sort of treatment have I/we been offered?

- What are the chances of success?
- How will the treatment change my life/our lives?
- How will I/we feel if the treatment does not succeed?
- How much do I/we want a child? How far am I/are we prepared to to to achieve parenthood?

and perhaps, most important of all

- Why do I/we want a child?

The answers which you give to these questions are vital to your decision-making process. The hard facts which you uncover can be discussed with a GP, obstetrician or a trained counsellor, and this should enable you to arrive at a good understanding of your chances of conceiving and giving birth to a healthy child. The British Infertility Counselling Association can put you in touch with someone who has been trained to help couples work through their infertility and sub-fertility problems, and ISSUE, the national organization for childless couples, produces a very useful series of leaflets about specific medical problems – as well as offering advice and support. The addresses of both organizations are given at the end of the book.

Of course, the issues are not simply factual. They are bound up with your own, and your partner's, emotional needs and desires – and these must also be talked through with someone you both trust implicitly to offer impartial advice and support. It is better to seek help from a trained counsellor rather than to rely on the advice of family or friends, who will be too close for the necessary impartiality and who won't have relevant information.

Your eventual choice must be based on a balance between facts and emotions. You may feel in your heart of hearts that you would do anything, pay any price – no matter how high – for the chance of a child. But if, *realistically*, your chances of achieving parenthood are minimal, is the risk worth taking? At what point will you decide to call it a day, and work on developing your life together as a childless couple? Will you be able to live with the pain when – after years of trying – you finally have to call a halt to your quest? At the other end of the spectrum, you may discover that your chances are really quite good; but decide to place a time-limit on fertility treatments in order to avoid exposing your relationship to additional strain.

Illness and disability

Parenting is hard work – ask any parent! It's not just the emotional and financial strains which children bring; bringing up children involves long hours and tough physical work, so it's certainly an advantage if you're in good shape before you start.

Some people feel that no price is too high to pay for a family of their own. Others decide that the physical stresses and strains would be just too much to bear. This is a particularly emotive question when the would-be parents are disabled, or suffer from a debilitating illness.

With support, physical disability need not be a barrier to parenthood, although there can be a whole host of practical problems. There have been many well-documented cases of severely disabled people making a great success of their families, even when both partners are handicapped. Disabled parenting does, however, require community support – and financial backing. Specially adapted accommodation and equipment may be required, and it may even be necessary to recruit additional professional help.

Some illnesses – like diabetes – need to be managed carefully, as if uncontrolled they can be damaging to the health of both mother and child during pregnancy. But the risks are relatively low if there is close medical supervision.

Other illnesses may not be life-threatening, and may even be regarded as trivial by society, but their impact upon the life of the mother may be so disabling that bearing and bringing up a child would be doubly difficult.

Tricia has two children aged five and two, and suffers from severe migraine, which she freely admits has a debilitating effect upon her life:

> People kept telling me that the attacks would go away if I got pregnant, so I suppose that hope was in the back of my mind when we decided to go ahead and have children. I've always had bad attacks – at least once a week, with severe vomiting and spots before the eyes, plus a really bad one around the time of my period, when all I can face doing is lying on the bed with the curtains drawn.
>
> I decided to have kids because not having them would be

like giving in to the migraine, admitting I was inferior to other people and couldn't cope with a normal life. I'd feel so ashamed. My mum had terrible headaches when I was a child, and she coped – so I reckoned I ought to be able to cope, too.

The migraines didn't get better – in fact they got worse. I went through my entire first pregnancy with a permanent headache, and I couldn't wait to get the birth over with. Since then, my attacks have more or less returned to the old pattern but I can't give in to them. When you've got a couple of young kids running around, you can't just crawl off to bed with a hot-water bottle and tell the world to go away! Some days, I feel so desperate. I just want to be alone with the pain, but I have to keep going for the children's sake. I do love my kids – love them more than anything – but I suppose I do wonder sometimes if I did the right thing. At the moment, they're too young to understand the pain. I keep on worrying that I'll pass the migraine on to them, too. It's not something I'd wish on anyone.

Ann is 35, married and was voluntarily sterilized six years ago. She had always vaguely assumed that she would have children, though she had no passionate feelings about motherhood. But a series of gynaecological problems left her with a tough decision to make:

> I had a bad fall which injured my back, and spent a long time in hospital, having surgery and convalescing. Afterwards, I knew my back was going to be weak and I'd have to take care of it. Anyhow, not long afterwards I started getting bad tummy and back pains and having trouble with incontinence, and it turned out that I'd got a prolapse. I had a couple of repair operations but nothing seemed to work – everything just came tumbling down again and the problems were as bad as ever.
>
> In the end, I'd had my cervix amputated and the doctors told me there was a strong chance I'd miscarry if I got pregnant. My husband and I had a long talk about everything, and discovered to our surprise that neither of us would be grief-stricken if we never became parents. It's funny, really. The final decision was really easy. We decided that, with my back problem and the worry about miscarriage,

trying for a baby just wasn't worth it. We talked over all the options with a counsellor, and I chose to be sterilized. From time to time I wonder what it might have been like having children, but I can honestly say I've never regretted our decision.

My husband always says that he married me for myself, not for my ability to have children. And he didn't want us to do anything that might risk my health. I think that's a wonderful way to feel. If anything, our decision has strengthened our relationship.

Sometimes, the desire for children can be so strong that emotion overrides medical advice. A recent newspaper story told of a professional woman in her 30s who was struck down with leukaemia just as she and her husband were deciding to start a family. The woman took the decision to postpone potentially life-saving treatment (which would make her sterile) until she had had time to try for a child. She now has her child but the new family faces an uncertain future, since if the treatment fails the mother has only an estimated two years to live.

Hereditary disorders

Despite the sophistication of modern medical science, hereditary genetic disorders such as cystic fibrosis and haemophilia remain a source of great tragedy. The sense of guilt and remorse can be overwhelming when parents discover that they have passed on a serious genetic disorder to their offspring – even when they had no idea that they were carriers.

If you are worried about a hereditary problem in your own or your partner's family, the best course of action is to ask your GP to refer you for genetic counselling. Counsellors are medically trained to examine the family history of both partners, looking for signs of possible hereditary disease, and calculating the risk that a disorder will be passed on.

Some disorders, such as glaucoma and Huntington's chorea, are carried in a dominant gene. This means that if only one of the partners carries the gene, the disorder can be passed on to the offspring. Recessive gene disorders, such as cystic fibrosis and phenylketonuria, can only be passed on if both partners carry the gene; and even then there is only a one-in-four chance that a child will be affected. Disorders which are linked to the x-chromosome (such as haemophilia and muscular dystrophy) are passed on through the female line, but the symptoms only manifest themselves in male children. Genetic counselling – although it cannot predict with absolute accuracy whether a child will be affected – can at least provide a balanced view of the risks involved, and help the prospective parents to come to a joint decision.

Of course, genetic counselling only provides you with the information to make your own decision; it cannot make your decision for you. Nor can it pinpoint those rare cases where a hereditary disorder appears spontaneously without any previous family history of the illness. Even if a risk has been identified, you may not necessarily decide to forget about having children. One man who suffers from brittle bone disease made a conscious decision to have a family, because he believed that despite the pain he had himself suffered his children would be able to live worthwhile and happy lives.

Doctors suspect that there may be a hereditary element in a host of other disorders, too, but in these cases the risks are much more difficult to calculate. Migraine and asthma are two of the illnesses which tend to 'run in families', and both can be very distressing for sufferers, despite modern medical treatments. Mental illnesses, such as schizophrenia and depression, may also be more likely to occur where there is an inbuilt predisposition to them.

Julia has no children, and freely admits to having no maternal 'instinct'. But if she had, she might well have decided not to have children because of the incidence of manic depression in her family – that is, if anyone had warned her of the dangers:

> Two years ago my mother killed herself in a hotel bedroom. She was 52 years old and had spent her entire adult life struggling against manic depression. During her last five years her condition gradually worsened, until towards the end she was constantly in and out of psychiatric hospitals, and her personality had undergone a complete change . . .
>
> As her only child I was naturally expected to look after my mother, during which time I spoke to many GPs and psychiatrists. None of these experts bothered to tell me that manic depression can be hereditary – I had to discover this for myself, and I am now reasonably sure that my grand-

mother, great grandfather and at least two other close relatives suffered from a milder form of the illness which eventually killed my mother.

British Organisation of Non-Parents (BON) Newsletter

Although it seems eminently sensible to consider the health and wellbeing of potential offspring, Julia feels that her views place her in a minority:

> So many people are so thoroughly brainwashed into the 'patter of tiny feet' mentality that they are quite prepared to play 'genetic roulette'. After all, life isn't complete without kids; who'll carry on the family name? Who's going to look after you in your old age? Insert your favourite cliché . . .

Birth defects

There are, of course, many non-genetic birth defects that can occur like cruel twists of fate. Heart defects, blindness, deafness, mental retardation, spina bifida and cerebral palsy can all transform the joy of birth into the anguished question: 'Why me?'

There is strong evidence that the mother's age is an important factor in the incidence of Down's Syndrome babies. For example, for mothers under 30, the chances of giving birth to a Down's child are very low – less than one in 2 000; but this figure rises to one in 280 for mothers aged 35–39, and becomes progressively higher as the mother's age increases. A mother aged 45 runs a one in 20 risk of giving birth to a Down's child.

Amniocentesis – a technique whereby a small sample of amniotic fluid (in which the fetus is bathed in the womb) is withdrawn and analysed – allows doctors to detect many serious illnesses and defects, including Down's Syndrome, before birth. However, it cannot be done before the mother is four months pregnant and carries a risk of causing a miscarriage. A new, safer test for Down's Syndrome has recently been developed at St Bartholomew's Hospital, and it is thought that the new test will be able to detect up to 60 per cent of cases – and at an early enough stage for the mother to have a termination – if that is what she wants.

All prospective parents worry about the health of their unborn children. Expectant mothers everywhere voice the same fears, the same hopes: 'As long as it's healthy, I'll be happy'. Although the risks to mother and child have been greatly reduced by developments in medical care, no one can guarantee that you will have a perfect, healthy child. But at least counselling is now available to help you take stock of the risk. At the end of the day, there are no easy answers. All you can do is look into your heart and ask yourself what is best for the child.

Questions for you and your partner:

- Is there a history of genetic disorders in my or your family?
- If so, what is the risk that your children will be affected?
- How old am I? Is there an age risk?
- How would I/we feel if I/we had a handicapped child?
- Would I/we be able to cope? And would I/we want to?
- How would you (the partner) feel? Would you be supportive?
- How much do I/we want a child?
- Why do I/we want a child?

Childless or child-free

We all feel the pressures upon us to have children – and yet some of us simply aren't cut out to be parents. Perhaps the single most common reason for not having children is personal preference: deciding that, for whatever reason, you would rather not become a parent. In fact, child-free living is a growing trend – so if you decide to pursue this course of action, you will not be alone – nor just part of a small cranky minority.

Recent statistics show that of all women born in 1955, around 17 per cent are still childless and say that they are 'not likely' to have children. This figure is expected to rise in the future, and it is quite possible that 19 or 20 per cent of today's 16-year-old girls will be childless. Many of these will be child-free by choice.

It is true that many people see having children as natural and inevitable – an essential part of the transition to adulthood and full membership of society. But parenthood is neither inevitable nor compulsory, since we now have access to highly effective methods of contraception.

Voluntarily child-free people are often the target of hostility and allegations of 'selfishness'. But an unwanted child can be an unhappy and disadvantaged child; and if the child-free are obeying selfish impulses in deciding not to have children, it seems a good deal more selfish to have a child as a designer fashion accessory, an insurance policy, a captive source of love or someone you can shape in your own image and send out into the world to do all the things you never quite got round to achieving!

Some people feel that they don't quite fit into the parental mould. They may be in happy marriages or other stable, loving relationships; but they just don't feel ready to bring another human being into their lives. They may have had an unhappy childhood, and be fearful of repeating the same mistakes with their own children as their parents made with them – something which psychologists recognize as an all-too-common reality. Or they may worry that they don't have the capacity to love a child, or to inspire love in return. And let's face it: not every woman has a maternal 'instinct', and not everyone enjoys the company of children.

The British Organisation of Non-Parents (BON) was founded in 1978, as a forum and information service for those who were not infertile, but had made a positive choice not to have children. Chairman Root Cartwright describes his own decision to be child-free:

> As far back as my early teens it was occurring to me that I would not want to have children. I couldn't imagine finding it acceptable to have my freedom of action circumscribed by family commitments, nor did I want to risk repeating the resentments and dishonesty which characterised my own childhood.
>
> *Liverpool Daily Post*, 18 September 1990

The fear of other people's hostility nudges many people into unwilling parenthood, but BON exists as a lifeline of reassurance for anyone considering a life without children.

BON member Myrna Hughes has been under pressure to procreate for most of her married life; she was born in Cyprus and her family and friends cannot understand her unwillingness to have children, even though Myrna, now 42, has a satisfying career as a solicitor.

> At first I procrastinated, said I didn't have any yet. Then I

would say I didn't want them. They would say: 'Never mind, there's time to change your mind'. People think I don't like children, it's not true. My brothers have kids and I love the role of an aunt. But I like giving them back at the end of the day. In the end it's my mother who suffers from the pressures more than me. People ask her all the time, at church and on the street, when will her daughter have children.

The Independent, 22 August 1990

Nevertheless, Myrna and her husband David are happy that they have made the correct decision, and they have no regrets or fears for the future.

Sally is also a BON member. She met her husband Steve nine years ago, and within a few days they had discovered that neither of them had ever wished to become a parent. For several years they used contraception, but when Sally developed problems with the Pill, they decided to take a more radical approach and Steve offered to have a vasectomy. Three years later, they are still happy with their choice.

Heather and Terry are both happy with their decision not to have children. When they met, three years ago, Terry already knew that he would not become a parent, as he had had a vasectomy six years previously, at the age of 26. Far from being dismayed, Heather was relieved:

> From being a little girl I've never had maternal instincts. And I remember hating the idea of being a housewife and mother. I always knew I wanted a career and children never came into that. I don't believe a woman has to have a child to be fulfilled. I have a wonderful relationship and I love my job. I'm as fulfilled as I could be.

Heather stresses that, far from setting the seal on their relationship, children would actually be detrimental to their happiness:

> The most important thing of all is that Terry and I really value our relationship. With children we wouldn't be able to spend as much quality time with each other. We don't need anyone else to enrich our relationship.

Daily Star, 6 March 1991

Sabine Hilgers is German but lives in Cambridge. She is disturbed by British reactions to the child-free:

> The problem is that over here it seems that everyone is so stereotyped. All the people in my age group (20–25) seem to want is to get engaged, get married and have their 2.7 children. All the people in my boyfriend's age group (30–37) have their mortgage and their kids and are not very stimulating either. I can't stand children, I never could, it was always clear to me that I would never have children, nor have I got the desire to get married.

She also refutes the popular belief that women who don't want children are career-oriented:

> The majority of people seem to think that when a couple don't want kids it must be because of career reasons. This is not true in our case. I only work part-time because I need a lot of time for myself and my interests and although I have a good position, I am anything but career-minded.
>
> BON Newsletter, January 1992

Of course, people's moods change and even the most dedicated non-parents can feel a twinge of regret when they are introduced to someone's well-behaved, intelligent, affectionate children.

Val is 33 and joined BON in 1991. She has made a decision not to have children, although she admits to having doubts and fears which many child-free people will identify with:

> I have been happily married for 11 years and I have never wanted children. I take a step away from babies, rather than towards them. I do not understand what makes people want children. My husband shares my views, but the situation for him is far more clear cut: there is no logical reason why we should have children and that's that. But seeing virtually all my otherwise normally sensible friends embarking on motherhood, I am afraid that at some dreadful moment I am going to be hit by whatever emotional or biological demand hit them.

Val is happy with her life, and cannot see how children would fit in. But her reasons also come from self-knowledge:

I don't think that I am 'parent material': I am not patient or practical, and though not a perfectionist I don't like doing things I am not good at. I am competitive and would find it difficult not to compete through my child. I have plenty of characteristics which I would not wish to pass on either by nature or nurture. It seems to me to take an astonishing degree of self-confidence verging on arrogance to embark on parenthood.

BON Newsletter, 1992

More and more people are questioning whether children would really bring them fulfilment, and this is surely a positive development. Modern parenting should be about positive choice, not about having children by accident, or as a way of being just like everybody else. Children are not in short supply in this overcrowded world. What's more, even in this relatively prosperous country, one in four children live on or below the European Community poverty line, and many more suffer because they have uncaring parents who abuse them or make them the scapegoats for their own problems and shortcomings. In unhappy relationships, it is often the innocent children who are used by their parents as ammunition in conflict.

Perhaps the worst scenario is when a couple decide to yield to pressure to have a child, only to discover after the birth that they have made a dreadful mistake. This happened to Hilary and Hugh:

Although pressure came mostly from Hilary's fears that she would have difficulty in conceiving, she and Hugh were led into a hasty decision which took no account of the fact that neither of them had ever had any positive urge to have children. Hilary even admits that she has always shied away from other people's babies, and felt awkward about touching them. But she made the mistake of thinking it would be different when she had her own child. Alas, once little Toby came along everything went horribly wrong:

At first I wondered if I was just suffering from postnatal depression. I didn't like Toby, I didn't like myself for having those feelings, and I resented Hugh for being able to get away from it all when he went to work.

Hugh, meanwhile, was feeling little better:

> I started to feel Toby was driving a wedge between us. I had already begun to think of our child as 'Him', because he seemed like a kind of monstrous shadow looming over our lives.

The couple have become gradually reconciled to their son's existence, but they still have mixed feelings. As Hugh explains:

> I cannot say that I love him in the way that I love Hilary . . . or that I know we were right to have a child. I would never say that to my family or even my friends. It sounds so unnatural and cruel. Perhaps there are simply some people who are not suited to parenthood, although it's possible my feelings will change as he grows up and becomes a proper person. All I can say is I sincerely hope so.
> 'First Person', *Marie Claire* magazine August 1992

The lesson of Hilary's story seems to be that you should never ignore any negative feelings you may have about parenthood. Unfortunately the tendency *is* to ignore them – because such feelings aren't acceptable. Sadly, therefore, there must be many other parents like Toby's, who still wonder if they made a mistake in having children.

At long last, there are those who are finally beginning to admit that they don't want to become parents. But it isn't enough just to want a child: you have to know *why* you want a child. Do you want it for the child's sake or for your own? Is it fair to have a child when you don't really like children? Only you can answer these questions – and it's important that you do.

Questions for you and your partner

- Have I/we ever felt a positive urge to have children? If not, why am I/are we considering having them now?
- When did I/we first begin to have doubts about having children? Have I/we always known that I/we didn't want children, or has the feeling developed recently, perhaps as a result of an identifiable event?
- Do I/we like children, and enjoy their company? If not, why am I/are we considering having them? Do I/we feel it is a duty,

or 'the thing to do'? Do I/we have enough experience of children to know if I/we really like them or not?
- If I was/we were told that I was/you were sterile, how would I/we feel? (devastated? relieved? cheated?)
- Would I/we have children to please someone else? (As we have seen, other people's wishes can sometimes make us do things we don't really want to do. Do I feel that I should please my partner by having children, even if I don't want them myself?)
- Why am I/are we considering having children? What do I/we think they will bring to my life/ our lives and our relationship? What do I/we think I/we have to offer them?
- Would I/we consider sterilization? If not, why not? Is it because our doubts have not yet crystallized into certainty?

The cost of parenthood

Make no mistake: having a child changes your life – forever. More so than marriage, parenthood is truly a lifetime commitment. The cost is more than just financial: having children takes a toll on emotions, relationships and every aspect of daily life. Parenthood can bring joys, tragedies, irritations and everyday pleasures, but one thing is for sure: once you have become a parent, there is no way that you will ever turn back your clock to the way you are now. So it's hardly surprising that not everyone is prepared to pay the price of parenthood.

FINANCIAL

Most young couples thinking of starting a family try to plan the births of their children so that the new family has a reasonably secure financial foundation. And it's true that the financial implications of having children should not be underestimated. Studies carried out by the Child Poverty Action Group and by university economists in Britain and America suggest that it costs somewhere between £45 000 and £60 000 to bring up a child to the age of 16. If the child goes to college and lives at home until he or she is 21, that figure could be around £100 000. Even spread out over a 20-year-period, that's a considerable sum of money.

Part of the financial cost of bringing up a child results from the effect on the mother's career. Except where the partner has a substantial income, most working women have to take some time out from their careers in order to care for their children. Many mothers are happy to do this, and share their child's early months or years and develop a strong bond of affection.

But it is worth setting aside the cuteness factor, and looking at the facts. According to Heather Joshi, an economist at London University, a woman who has two children may lose nine or ten years of full employment, while the loss may be up to 20 years if she returns only to part-time work. Based on 1986 figures, this would represent a loss of earnings of somewhere around £122 000 for a woman earning only £6 000 per annum, and who has only one child. For a woman on a high salary, and with two or more children, the figures are clearly even more depressing. On the other hand, experts estimate that the cost of having the first child is about three times as high as the cost of having any subsequent children.

Money isn't everything, of course. But for most of us, waiting until we could afford to have a child would mean waiting for ever. Most people who have children do manage to cope financially, though they have to make certain sacrifices. However, not having enough money can put an enormous strain on relationships, and the unpalatable truth is that, the more financially secure you are, the easier it is to enjoy being a parent.

Questions for you and your partner:

- How financially secure am I/are we?
- What would be the financial effects of having a child?
- Would I/we have to continue working after the birth? If so, how would I/we feel about this?
- How important is money to me/us?
- How do I/we feel about a reduction in my/our standard of living?
- If I/we waited a while, would the financial impact be less severe, or worse?

CHANGING RELATIONSHIPS AND LIFESTYLES

It's a dreadful mistake to assume that you can have a child and carry on with your life in exactly the same way. The harsh realities of parenthood are not just confined to the agony of the monthly bank statement. Having children brings irreversible changes in lifestyle, career and relationships.

Babies are not babies for long. They don't stay as cute,

immobile little bundles for more than a few months. Very rapidly, they begin to assert themselves as separate human beings, with their own right to existence. Once you have spent a few sleepless nights attending to your child's needs, you realize that you and your partner are now sharing each other with a third – and maybe a fourth or fifth – person. The change from being lovers to being Mum and Dad can take quite some getting used to. Inevitably, adjustments must be made; and relationships must change.

Motherhood can be an intensely isolating experience after the expectation and attention lavished upon the mother-to-be during her pregnancy. Suddenly the fuss is all over. The doctors and midwives and friends and relations have all gone away, and the new mother is left alone to look after her baby. After a life of independence, she finds that she is suddenly marooned in the house, staring at four walls, unable to go out when and where she pleases. This isolation can be terrifying, particularly as so few women have contact with young children before they give birth to their own, and they may have no one to turn to for support or advice.

The relationship between partners changes, as man and woman have to adjust to their new roles as mother and father. In her book, *Mad to be a Mother*, Brigid McConville includes a vivid evocation of the impact of these shifting perceptions upon the new father, who may view the new relationship between mother and child with jealousy:

> Perhaps he loves her for the freedom of her spirit, for the beauty of her body? How ironic then that the product of his love – their child – should so deeply jeopardize her autonomy and change her body irrevocably. He thought he had secured first place in her affections, only to be usurped by a tiny tyrant whom he cannot fight. Now he lies in bed beside his woman, watching his baby suck on the breasts that he had thought of as his preserve.

Friendships also change, particularly between the new mother and her childless friends. The childless woman may feel a sense of betrayal as she sees all her friends moving into motherhood, drawing away from her into a new-found world which by its very nature excludes those without children. She may even feel that her friend has 'sold out', forfeited the right to respect because she has given up her place in the competitive world of work.

New mothers can also appear thoroughly self-absorbed and inward-looking, so wrapped up in their children that they have only one topic of conversation. The isolation restricts their experience of the world. Where once they would talk about work, hobbies, books they had read and plays they had seen, they now talk about their children – and little else. Motherhood is exhausting as well as satisfying, and it is extremely difficult to maintain the outside interests which were once so important. So it's no great surprise that many old friendships cool off – simply because the childless woman and the new mother no longer have anything to talk about – or indeed the opportunity to meet!

Of course, many mothers (and fathers) would say that these drawbacks are a small price to pay for the joy which their children have brought them. The infant stage doesn't last for ever, and within a few years some of the strands of social life and careers can begin to be picked up again. But life can never be exactly as it was before.

It all comes down to the cost of choosing. Every choice you make has a cost. As Renate Olins of London Marriage Guidance points out: 'If you have the red dress, you can't have the blue one. You can't have absolutely everything. There are always losses.' For both parents, there is a high cost to pay in terms of loss of freedom and autonomy. For the mother, there may also be a permanent impact in career terms:

> If you give up work to have children, very few women get back to the same level. They may never achieve what they would have achieved.

And yet, with more than one in every three marriages ending in divorce, now is the time when women need to safeguard their careers, in case they are left, literally, holding the baby. For some women, the price may simply be too high.

Questions for you and your partner:

- What impact do I/we think children would have on my/our lifestyle?
- Am I/are we prepared for change?
- How do I/you feel about change?

Ideological considerations

World resources are finite, and the environment has already been seriously damaged – primarily by the demands of industrialized Western societies, and the harmful by-products of our factories, cars and intensive agriculture. Yet we in the West continue to press for population control in Third World nations (whose people often have ecologically sustainable lifestyles) whilst failing to address the problem in our own countries. The Green movement aims to encourage everyone to limit the size of their families, particularly in industrialized societies which use up the highest proportion of world resources.

Occasionally, an individual or couple decides against parenthood for ideological reasons. This trend has begun to take off with the growing popularity of the 'Green' movement which encourages families to consider having either no children or just one. Experts agree that the world is already in the middle of a terrible population crisis, and it has been suggested that the population of the UK should be reduced to 30 or 40 million.

Angela is a member of the Green Party, and in her mid-30s. At the age of eleven, she decided not to have children because she was already very concerned about the environment, and admits that she 'did not think it a great sacrifice'. She explains her decision:

> My main reason for deciding not to have children was environmental, as I believe that the world is over-populated. It seemed a logical thing for me not to have children. Moreover, women without children seem to be happier and lead fuller lives.

Friends, relatives and colleagues have generally been supportive of Angela's decision, although:

> The husband of one friend horrified me by saying I ought to have children as I was white. Some work colleagues have found it hard to believe I did not want children. A male colleague – when I asked him what he thought I ought to do after I got my Open University degree – suggested I should have a baby!

Angela occasionally feels a sense of regret, but concludes that her choice was the right one – not only for the environment, but for her own needs. She has:

> freedom to go to the pub, travel abroad, and spend time and money on studying, charities and politics. I feel that having children has to mean changes in lifestyle for most women in our present society and that very few manage to combine a career as opposed to a job with having children. I'm afraid I cannot think of any bad things about being child-free except the tendency to be smug and self-satisfied with my chosen lifestyle.

Questions for you and your partner:

- Do I/we have any beliefs which would conflict with a desire to have children?
- If so, do they outweigh the desire for children?
- Would I/we rather limit the size of my/our family, or have no children at all?

Single parenting

These days, around one in every five children is born to an unmarried woman. True, many of these mothers are in stable relationships with a live-in boyfriend, whilst others are separated or divorced. But a significant proportion of today's new mothers are, and intend to remain, single. Some single men are becoming parents, too: either looking after their own children after a separation or the death of the mother, or becoming foster or adoptive parents in their own right.

Having a child whilst leading a single life is much more feasible today than it used to be; but that doesn't mean it is easy. Being a single parent means being both father and mother to a child, and carrying all the responsibilities on your shoulders alone. If you are thinking of single parenting, you will need great reserves of physical and emotional strength, a well-developed sense of humour and a talent for problem-solving – not to mention a degree of financial security that will give both you and your child a good start and help reduce some of your worries to manageable proportions.

Single parenting can also entail complex adult relationships. What if you aren't on good terms with the other parent? He or she may well be granted reasonable access to the child, even if you aren't on speaking terms, or if the other parent has had nothing to do with the child since its conception.

Having a small child in tow can also play havoc with your other relationships, both with friends and lovers who may not want to be involved in the nappy-changing rituals of parenthood.

There are bound to be lots of practical problems, too. If you are caring for a child on your own, you will feel obliged to work hard to support both of you and to give your child some of the luxuries which you would like to provide. But if you are out at work all day, who is going to care for your child? You are going to need watertight childcare arrangements which will not have you constantly in tears, worrying how you are ever going to succeed in juggling parenthood with your career. Perhaps you have a helpful relative or know another single mum who would be willing to help out. Even so, prepare yourself for emotional upset as you feel pulled in two (or all!) directions.

If you have a busy job, you are bound to arrive home sometimes feeling tired and irritable. But you must then start on your other 'career' – caring for your child, who has not seen you all day and who naturally wants to play and chatter and be cuddled by you – just as you want to chatter and cuddle, if only you didn't feel so tired! Some single parents find it all too much to cope with as the conflicts breed resentment, and opt either for part-time work or for staying at home until the child goes to school.

Having a child is always a big step to take, even when the child will have two parents who are equally committed to his/her wellbeing. On the plus side, however, research studies do show that children are far better off with one, loving parent than they would be if their parents lived together in an unhappy relationship. Single parents can, and do, bring up happy, well-balanced children in a loving home environment, but don't underestimate the importance of motivation, planning and determination.

The second time around

Many relationships breakdown these days, and it is not uncommon for people to have second families. Indeed, there is often much soul-searching about whether or not to embark on parenthood second time around. The question can be especially emotive if one partner has never had children before and the other has a grown-up family. Not everyone wants to go through the noise and disruption of a young family for a second time – especially in 'middle' age. Other people, though, gain a whole new lease of life from second-time parenting. One thing is for sure: it's a question that needs thrashing out before partners make a commitment to each other. It is not a light issue, and if unresolved it could cause much heartache and discord later on.

When Pam met her husband Roy, it didn't seem to matter that the divorced father of two had had a vasectomy. But Pam was 24 years younger than Roy, and after a few years she started to feel 'broody'. They discussed vasectomy reversal, but Roy said he was not ready for it. Pam began to get worried:

> At one stage, I thought that we would never have children and for a period of about six months I was very depressed. It was obvious that if we did not have children it would be a problem. I never got to the stage of feeling resentful. But I would have done, I'm sure, if Roy hadn't had the reversal. I think we both realized that, although it wasn't his fault, he was, in effect, preventing me from having a baby.

Roy slowly realized that he would have to consider having the reversal, and over a period of time he came to the conclusion that he positively wanted to have children with Pam. He had the vasectomy reversal, and – although he wasn't optimistic about the chances of success – a few months later Pam conceived.

Fortunately, both Pam and Roy are delighted with their new family and have no regrets. Roy has found that his relationship with his other two children has improved since the birth of baby Nic. But what would have happened if Roy had not had a change of heart? Pam admits: 'I can't tell whether we would have stayed together'.

Kilroy's Casebook

Yvonne met Malcolm in mid-life, after an unhappy first marriage as a result of which she left her four-year-old twins with their father. She made it clear to Malcolm from the start that she did not want any more children and – although he had not been married before – he understood this clearly, and told her that he had no burning desire to be a father.

Yvonne acknowledges that her original reasons for having children were unwise:

> I had an unhappy, disturbing childhood which I've only in the last five years begun to acknowledge. I thought that having my own children would alleviate the pain of my childhood, but in fact it made the pain sharper. I felt very much a child, and needed to learn to mother and father myself, a skill I've learned quite well over the years. I'm very much an individual and I felt overwhelmed by the loss of my identity and the new identity of 'mother'.

Before her first marriage, Yvonne told her husband that she did not want children; but it later transpired that he felt that having no children . . .

> put a question mark over his manhood. He was threatened by my wanting to be different from my peers, and also found it threatening to live with a career-minded wife. The marriage would not have lasted without children and didn't survive with them – there's a moral there somewhere.

When it came to making the decision with Malcolm, Yvonne was quite certain that she did not want to have any more children:

> I love my children dearly and felt that if I had any more children, it would be seen as the ultimate rejection of them. I had left them, that was bad enough, but to replace them with another child – well! Both of my children (one male, one female) have in the last year said the fact that Malcolm and I had no babies helped them come to terms with losing me.

Some people have accused Yvonne and Malcolm of being selfish in not having children, but Yvonne's twins spend each school holiday with them, and she is 'not sure about the selfishness'. Although Yvonne is a teacher and is experienced with maladjusted children, she has had 'no inclination to reproduce'.

Questions for you and your partner:

- Do I/we positively want a second family?
- How do I/we feel about bowing to your/each other's wishes?

- Could I resent my/our new family or my partner/each other?
- How do I/we feel about being an 'elderly' parent?
- What do I/we think children would add to our relationship?

Summary

As we have seen, there are all sorts of problem issues which need to be discussed and resolved before a sensible, informed decision can be made. For some people, the decision-making process will be long and arduous: but there is arguably no more important issue to resolve than that of whether or not to have children.

In the next chapter, we shall be looking in more detail about the questions which all prospective parents should ask themselves, and guiding you through the decision-making process towards the solution which is right for you.

4
Making Your Decision

Unlike other major life decisions (e.g. getting married, living together), it is impossible to try out parenthood in advance to see if it suits you. There is no opportunity to get to know your child before it is born – and once he or she is born, there is inevitably no going back. This makes the decision a very difficult one to make. Since it is supposedly a free choice, the responsibility for getting it right is yours and yours alone – and that is quite a frightening thought.

This chapter addresses the major issues which you (and your partner) should consider before embarking on parenthood. At the end of the chapter are questions to help in the decision-making process. These are based on leaflets supplied by the British Organization of Non-Parents (BON) which has a great deal of experience in helping individuals and couples through their decision-making process. Their address is given at the end of the book for further information.

Choice and 'decidophobia'

One of the problems about deciding whether or not to have a child is the fact that, until very recently, it was not considered to be a real decision. Most women chose to marry, and once married were expected to have children. A married woman without children was automatically regarded with pity. Contraception was unreliable and regarded with suspicion, so there was little hope for the couple who did not want children.

The advent of the Pill in the late 1960s brought a new freedom of choice for women: the ability to choose when, and whether, their children would be born. The legalization of abortion both extended this freedom of choice and reduced the numbers of babies available for adoption. This meant that more women than ever before would remain child-free.

It is only very recently that the deliberate choice not to have children has begun to gain respectability. There are a host of reasons for making the choice not to have children: the planet is overcrowded, more and more women are choosing to find fulfilment in their careers, rather than in motherhood, and not everyone is Superwoman, capable of combining the two – not everyone wants to; couples may feel that the closeness of their relationship might suffer if they became parents.

Of course, most people do ultimately want to become parents. But there are many who are undecided, and put off making the decision because they shun the responsibility and are afraid of the consequences.

WHO MAKES THE DECISION?

Very often, 'decidophobia' eventually leads to a choice being made without any *conscious* decision having been made. Research suggests that perhaps as many as two in every three pregnancies within marriage are unplanned. Couples, unable to make a firm decision for or against, end up taking inadequate (or no) contraceptive precautions and the rest is left to chance.

Studies of problem children have suggested that a higher than average proportion of them were born from unplanned or unwanted pregnancies. Also parents who have experienced unwanted pregnancy are more likely than other couples to have marital problems, and their divorce rates are higher too.

It seems very sad that so many children should be born by accident, simply because their parents are bad decision-makers. What's more, 'decidophobia' often only affects one of the prospective parents, whilst the other holds strong and uncompromising views, for or against. Take the example of Margaret and Gary. Margaret explains:

> We got married because we wanted to be together. I'd never really thought much about having kids, and I didn't have any strong views for or against. But I soon realized that Gary badly wanted kids, and couldn't understand why I didn't feel as strongly as he did. In the end, I just went along with what he wanted because I loved him and I didn't want to hurt him or do anything which might damage our relationship. We had two kids in four years. Now, when I look back on it, I'm not so sure we did the right thing. I had to give up my job (which I really enjoyed) and I'm beginning to wonder if we shouldn't have talked it over a bit more before we took the plunge.

Andrea wanted children very much, and persuaded her husband Ray to go along with her wishes, although she knew that he was not enthusiastic about becoming a parent. Since the birth of their daughter, Emily, she has deeply regretted forcing him into fatherhood. Ray refuses to assume any responsibility at all for Emily, and her teachers have noticed that she seems withdrawn and unhappy at school. According to Andrea:

> Whenever Emily has a problem, or one of her frequent temper tantrums, Ray insists on calling her 'your daughter' or even 'your mistake' when he speaks to me. I'd hoped that after all these years he'd have let byegones be byegones.

David and Myrna are members of the British Organization of Non-Parents (BON), although David has two children from a previous marriage. David suffered badly from asthma as a child, and did not want to risk passing on the problem to his own children. But his first wife felt very differently:

> ...Her distress was palpable: she had always wanted children, family pressures were high, the social norm was (and is) not to heed these things. Science would provide an answer. I gave in.
> We had two children, now attractive, intelligent young adults: a source of great pleasure and pride to a loving father. But my daughter is mildly asthmatic, and my son may well be carrying the genes to hand on to his children (if any).
> ...When I look at my daughter I cannot imagine life without her, but still I think I was wrong to concede on a matter about which I felt passionately. I sacrificed my principles. I did so because I felt guilty that my views caused distress, and because the social pressures on my wife caused secondary pressure on me. There is no comfort in the thought that in one way I acted unselfishly in following the views of others. How many potentially child-free couples do exactly that?

A great deal of distress and conflict can arise when partners do not discuss the issue of childbearing and come to a compromise which is acceptable to both of them. Obviously this is an emotive subject, and not one which lends itself to purely logical argument. The impulse to have children is never purely logical: it is bound up with emotions and gut-reactions and philosophical convictions which another person may find difficult to understand and accept, and influenced by expectations and assumptions that few of us ever question.

Nevertheless, if you are in a stable one-to-one relationship and considering whether or not to have a child, it is essential to discuss the matter between you at length, and to make sure – as far as one ever can be: there are *no* guarantees or absolutes – that your eventual decision is the right one for both of you.

Talk about the consequences of having a child which your partner does not want. He or she might refuse to take any part in its upbringing, or to show it any affection. Such behaviour would be bound to damage the child (as well as your own relationship with your partner). It's not good enough simply to have a child because *you* want one, and shrug your shoulders and say: 'Never mind; he/she will come round in the end'.

Equally important, it is unwise to allow the decision to be made for you by someone else, whether parents, friends or the media – although, as we have seen, these are all very persuasive and real pressures.

Parents often hanker after grandchildren, for many reasons – not least perhaps, as a way of enjoying all the pleasant aspects of parenthood and avoiding the unpleasant ones. But they can cause dreadful feelings of guilt, as BON member Gill Taylor explains:

> Being an only child, I know that I've deprived my parents of their grandchildren ... My husband and I used to get hints from them but now they've come to terms with it. But I do feel guilty and isolated at times. I wonder if I'm selfish not to want to sacrifice my life to bring up another person.

Friends and acquaintances can put the pressure on too. Even if you don't have a particularly strong maternal drive, it's hard to look at your pregnant peers with their toddlers, and listen to their constant exhortations to 'join the club'. It's so much easier to conform than to do what you really want to do.

Meanwhile, media stereotypes of perfect motherhood only add to the pressure, and certainly don't make decisions any easier to take. Women's magazines in particular have a lot to answer for: it's easy for people with little real experience of babies and children (and this is the case for most young adults these days,) to be brainwashed into thinking that the whole process will be a sort of Laura Ashley dream: clean and bright and frilly and laundered and predictable.

In the final analysis, any decision you make has to be *yours*. If you're a single woman, then it must be your decision, ideally in conjunction with the prospective father. If you're half of a couple, then the two of you must decide together. Which doesn't of course mean that you can't take advice, or discuss the matter with others, too. We all need to learn how to refuse to give in to other people's selfish pressures, to listen to our hearts, and to weigh up the pros and cons of any advice we are given.

Whatever the decision you make, there must be a positive decision: you owe that much both to yourselves and to your future children. If you are thinking of getting married, or 'settling down', it is much better for you and your partner to sort out your feelings about children beforehand.

The decision-making process

Much of the information which follows is adapted from leaflets produced by the British Organization of Non-Parents (BON), a support group which aims to promote the responsibility of choice in childbearing.

WOULD YOU MAKE A GOOD PARENT?

As we have seen, most people approach the question of childbearing with rather less care than they would invest in choosing a new vacuum cleaner. There is a tendency to assume that children will come along some time, or that there will be plenty of time to make a decision. Few people ask themselves if they would make good parents, and for most, the vague desire to have a baby (for whatever reason) is sufficient to add one or two more new human beings to the 5 billion or so currently inhabiting the Earth.

One of the major factors in successful parenting seems to be the parents' own experience during childhood. If we feel as if our own parents did a reasonable job of bringing us up; if we have happy memories of our childhood and an affectionate relationship with our parents, there seems to be a pretty fair chance that we will be good parents too and able, and willing to meet our child's many needs. But those who suffered a deprived or unhappy childhood may (but only may) find they still have a core of yearning and unmet needs left over from childhood which would interfere with their being able to give and meet their own children's needs and make them happy. In such cases, it may be a good idea to have some counselling before gaining experience of being with babies and children, to gain confidence with them and find out if you are happy in their company and want to spend more time with them. But be warned; being with children will put you in touch with your own childhood feelings and experiences – which, if not happy, can be painful and make you want to distance yourself from your child as you want to distance yourself from your past. There is nothing *wrong* about not liking children, or not wanting to be a parent. What *is* wrong is not knowing yourself and bringing unwanted children into the world just because it seemed a nice idea, to please other people or to conform to some fatuous social norm.

Having children is a stressful experience. It requires a certain skill in interpersonal relationships, lots of tolerance and vast amounts of motivation.

Here are some questions for you and your partner to ask yourselves:

- Do I/we like children?
- How strongly do I/we feel about having children?
- Did I/we have a good relationship with my/our parents when a child? What is that relationship like now? Would I/we want a similar relationship with my/our own children?
- Have I/we had much contact with babies, toddlers, teenagers (e.g. babysitting, teaching, youth work, friends' or relatives' children)?
- Would I/we find it easy to feel affection towards a child?
- How much affection would I/we expect to receive from my/our child?
- Am I/are we patient and tolerant?
- Can I/we cope with noise, disruption, confusion, inconvenience?
- Could I/we cope with moody teenagers?
- Can I/we control my/our anger? Might I/we lose my/our temper(s) and become violent towards my/our child?
- Could I/we cope with the issues of freedom and discipline, without becoming too strict or too easygoing?
- Would I/we worry about my/our child, and become overprotective?

- Could I/we cope if things weren't perfect?
- What if my/our decision to have a child turned out to have been wrong for me/us?

There are no 'right' and 'wrong' answers to questions like those listed above. They are simply there to help you think clearly about the issues involved, and arrive at a joint decision which is right for you.

WOULD A CHILD FIT INTO YOUR WAY OF LIFE?

For many people, a child is seen as an essential part of marriage: representing the transition from newly-wed couple to new family unit. Yet a growing number of married, and unmarried, couples feel that children are not necessary for their happiness and fulfilment, particularly where both partners have demanding jobs or many outside interests, or where a female partner is keen to carry on with her career.

There is no doubt that having a child implies accepting considerable disruption. Life is never quite the same again once you have had a baby. It's not just the sleepless nights in the first few months: it's the realization that you have made a lifelong commitment.

You will have to support your child at least up to the age of 16, and quite possibly until he or she has finished a college education. And what parent stops worrying about a child just because he or she has reached 18 or 21? The commitment to a child is very much a commitment for life. If you have two or three children, with a two or three year age-gap between them, you will have teenagers at home well into your middle years, particularly if – like many people nowadays – you postpone having children until you are in your 30s.

Particularly during the first months of a baby's life, parents can experience considerable problems as they battle to cope not only with the demands of the child, but with the sudden restriction of their own activities. They realize that they are no longer free to do exactly what they want. Mothers who stay at home to look after their children may feel depressed because they rarely get out, and couples will find their social life severely restricted – it's difficult to accept last-minute invitations, or decide to go out on a whim, because reliable babysitters are thin on the ground and very much in demand. But on the plus-side is the effect children can have on you – if you let them. After all, parenting involves dynamic interraction and a child can teach you a great deal; you can change, evolve, mature in a way that is probably unique to parenting because a child can get to those parts of you that are well hidden from adults.

Not least in importance are the financial considerations. It is not so much a question of asking: 'Can I afford a child?' as asking if a child is your first priority. Most people can manage financially if they have to, but not everyone wants to, and introducing a child into a situation of financial diffiulty is likely to provoke resentments between parents, and towards the child.

Ask yourselves these questions:

- Would having a baby interfere with my/our education, training or careers? If so, could I/we cope with this? Could I/we postpone my/our plans, or fit them in with bringing up a child?
- Would I/we have to give up interests and activities which I/we feel are important?
- If I/we plan to combine having children with continuing to work, can I/we cope? Do I/we have the necessary energy in the evenings, after a hard day at work? What about working part-time?
- Can I/we cope financially? Currently, it costs an estimated £80 per week to bring up a child, and I/we will be committed financially at least until the child is 16.
- Do I/we live in an area where I/we would like to bring up a child? If not, would I/we be willing and able to move?
- Am I/are we willing to accept restrictions on my/our social life, leisure time and privacy?
- Would I/we have a baby to prove to others that I/we had grown up (though, of course, such a motive would indicate the opposite)?
- Would I/we have a baby to feel that I/we 'fitted in' with others of my/our age?
- Would I/we have a baby so that my/your/our parents could become grandparents?
- Would I/we have a baby because I was/we were bored or dissatisfied with my life/our lives and/or career(s), and wanted to 'opt out'? (It is belatedy being acknowledged that for many women having children is the soft option: despite sleepless

nights etc., they opt out of the economic struggle and became dependent upon partner, state or paid help.)
- Would I/we have a baby as an excuse to work part-time?
- Would I/we have a baby as an attempt to 'heal' a bad relationship?
- If I/we didn't have any children, do I/we think I/we would feel unfulfilled? If so, why?
- If I/we had a child, would I/we want it to be like me/us/you?
- How would I/we feel about adopting a child?
- How would I/we feel if my/our child grew up to have ideas and beliefs which were radically different from my/our own?
- Would I/we expect my/our child to do all the things I/we wished I/we had done?
- Am I/are we happy to devote at least 16 years of my life/our lives, to being responsible for my/our child?
- If your partner died, or left you, would you be able to cope as a single parent?
- If I am contemplating single or gay parenthood, or have a disability, am I/are we sure that I/we can cope with the practical implications and will be able to provide a happy and secure environment for a child to grow up in?
- If I/we have a child and place it with a child-minder when s/he is a few months old, what is the nature of my/our relationship with the child other than one of 'ownership'?

WHY DO YOU WANT TO HAVE A CHILD?

Obviously, having a child is more than just a case of considering the practical implications. One of the major considerations is whether or not you and your partner actually want children – and are not just thinking of having them to please somebody else, or to escape the overwhelming pressures which society places upon childless couples and individuals.

But it isn't enough just to know that you want children: you must also think carefully about *why* you want them. For surely the most important consideration is that the child's interests must come first. And if you are having children for a selfish reason, or to please your parents or friends, you should realize that these are hardly good enough reasons for doing anything – let alone bringing a new person into the world.

Ask yourselves these questions:

- Would I/we expect my/our child to look after me/us in old age? If so, why?
- Do I/we think I/we need to have a baby to make my/our marriage complete? If so, why?
- Do I/we want a child to give me/us something to love, and something which will love me/us in return? If so, is it possible to find this love in any other way, and from any other source? How can I/we assume that the relationship will be positive?
- Would I/we feel strongly about wanting either a boy or a girl? Why? And what if I/we didn't get the one I/we wanted?
- Do I/we want to have a child? If so, why?

Perhaps you have discovered that your reasons for wanting to have a family are not quite what you thought they were. As we saw earlier on in the book, there is still a lot of debate about whether or not the desire for children is mainly a biological drive or one which society fosters through environment and upbringing. Without a doubt, many women do experience strong maternal feelings and respond very positively to small babies. Many men also feel that they would like the chance to love and nurture a new human being. On the other hand, babies do not remain babies for long. They soon outgrow the cute and cuddly stage, and become egocentric, demanding toddlers – and later adolescents – stretching even the most devoted parent's patience. There seems little wisdom in giving into the drive to procreate if you only like small babies.

Also, it is definitely not a good idea to have a child as an attempt to cement a flagging relationship. A child is a challenge to a relationship and in most cases, the birth of a baby will undermine an ailing ménage, and the child ends up the victim of a broken home.

Last but not least, you need to explore the possibility that you are having a baby as an excuse to avoid making other decisions about your life: for example, career choices, choices about problems in your relationship.

ARE YOU AND YOUR PARTNER IN AGREEMENT?
Having a child needs to be a joint decision. You and your partner will be taking on the greatest responsibility of your lives – one which will change your way of life beyond recognition. And this new member of your family needs to be welcomed by both of you.

Ask yourselves these questions:

- Do we both feel equally positive about having a child?
- How would we feel if one of us said that he or she did not want a child? Would we feel rejected? Would we try to change his or her mind?
- Would we still see our relationship as a lifelong one, if our partner did not want children?
- How would we manage the conflict? Do we feel that our relationship is strong enough to withstand it?
- What would we do – would we consider having a child, even if one of us did not want one?
- Are we happy together, and do we think we could provide a child with a happy home?
- If we had a child and later encountered insoluble problems, would we be able to separate? Or would we feel obliged to stay together for the sake of the child? How could we know which would actually be better for the child?
- Would we be able to share each other with a baby without jealousy?
- How do we feel about bringing a child into an overpopulated world with many social and environmental problems?
- Are there any special difficulties (e.g. medical conditions) which might influence our decision for or against having children? If so, are we prepared to undergo appropriate counselling and carry out the recommendations?
- How many children do we want, and how are we going to space them out? What methods of family planning should we be using?
- If one of us wants a child, and the other doesn't, what do we do?

CAN YOU MEET A CHILD'S NEEDS?

Human beings have three main sorts of needs: physical, intellectual and emotional – all of which must be met if that person is going to be a happy, safe and well-balanced individual.

The NSPCC has identified 10 basic needs which all children have. Read through the list below (adapted from the NSPCC booklet, *Understanding Children Better*) and ask yourselves if you could meet all of these needs – not just now, but throughout the time the child will be dependent on you:

- Basic physical care (warmth, shelter, food and rest, hygiene, medical care etc.)
- Love and affection (including cuddles and comforting)
- Security (continuity of care, daily routines, a secure family group, consistent rules)
- Stimulation and teaching (to help the child achieve its full potential and explore the world)
- Guidance and control (to teach sociable behaviour)
- Responsibility (giving the child opportunities and encouragement in learning to look after him/herself and making decisions, making mistakes and learning from them)
- Independence (helping the child to learn decision-making in a protected environment)
- Actively promoting the child's self-esteem (showing pride and pleasure, interest and delight in what the child is doing, so that the child feels good about him/herself)
- Approval (making allowances, showing admiration, spending time together as companions)
- Promoting general emotional health (through supporting and caring, comforting, helping the child to deal with pain and loss, and helping introduce the concept of life as joyful and worthwhile).

Your decision

Parenthood isn't just a case of making a straightforward decision: shall I or shan't I have children? It means taking into account all the factors discussed above, so that you and your partner can decide:

- Do we want children at all?
- If we do, do we want them now, or shall we wait?
- How long should we wait?
- If there are genetic or other problems and the fetus is diagnosed abnormal, are we prepared to consider abortion? If not, can we cope with a disadvantaged child?
- How many children should we have?
- How big a space should we leave between them?

Summary

In the final analysis, no one can tell you whether or not you ought to have children; and no one can look into your heart and tell how much you want to have them. The decision has to be yours, and your partner's.

On the other hand, careful thought and extensive discussion can help avoid some of the serious pitfalls of unplanned parenthood. Of course, you'll probably still make mistakes: no one can predict how well parenthood will work out. But at least talking things through thoroughly beforehand will help you stand the best chance of making the *right* decision for you. Bringing a child into the world is an irrevocable act. Equally, male and female sterilization are essentially irreversible. Once you make your decision, you'll have to stick to it – so it makes sense to try and ensure it's the right one for you.

Perhaps you are fond of children, but feel that having your own birth-children is not the right option for you. In the next chapter, we look at two of the alternatives to biological parenting: fostering and adoption.

5
Alternatives to Childbearing

Adoption and fostering are often seen as the province of the infertile – the only alternatives for those who want to become biological parents, but cannot. In this respect, adopting a child can sometimes seem like 'second best': something that you only consider doing if there is no other way of becoming a parent. While it is true that adoption and fostering do offer a lifeline to infertile couples and individuals, they are by no means their exclusive prerogative. An increasing number of single people are looking for new ways of parenting, and some couples are turning to fostering and adoption as a preferred alternative to childbearing.

Adoption

Traditionally, childless couples have looked to adoption agencies to provide a solution to their desire for parenthood. But the number of children available for adoption has been falling consistently in recent years, and adoption agencies have very stringent criteria which anyone who wishes to become an adoptive parent must fulfil.

WHAT IS ADOPTION? THE FACTS
Adopting a child means welcoming him or her into your home and taking on the role of parent. It is a lifelong commitment – unlike fostering, which is generally short-term. The responsibilities are exactly the same as those you would have if you were the child's natural parents.

Children available for adoption
When people first consider adopting a child, they often think in terms of adopting a 'normal, healthy' baby. Not so very long ago, this was a realistic ambition, and some adoptive parents were even able to choose the sex and appearance of the child. These days, however, with contraception, abortion and changing attitudes to single-parent families, there are very few 'healthy' babies available for adoption.

Some people are able to adopt *babies*, but they are the exceptionally lucky ones. Normally you would need to be within a certain age range (up to 32 or 40, depending on the local age requirements) and fulfil many other requirements. However, there are thousands of other children who *desperately* need to find permanent new families. These children are said largely to have 'special needs', meaning any of the following:

- children with physical disabilities or illnesses
- the children of HIV-positive parents
- children with mental disabilities
- children who need to be placed with parents of a particular ethnic origin
- older children
- brothers and sisters who need to stay together.

Obviously, caring for a child with special needs requires special qualities. You need to be patient, understanding, energetic and totally committed. And of course, you must enjoy being with children, and with your child in particular.

Adopting children from abroad
Recently, the television and newspapers have been bombarding us with pictures of children in countries like Romania and Bosnia. These children are unwanted and uncared-for, suffer from terrible physical and emotional deprivation, and desperately need a loving, secure home with warmth, food and lots of love and cuddles.

It is very easy to see these pictures and think: 'Why don't we adopt a child from abroad?' But in practice adopting children from other countries is very difficult, expensive, time-consuming, and – in the long run – may not be in the best interests of the child. Many experts believe that it is best if children keep in touch with their own ethnic background, rather than being brought into a new country, where they may grow up to feel like strangers.

There are no adoption agencies in Britain that help people to adopt children from overseas. So if you are keen to pursue this course of action you will need to make all the necessary arrangements with the DSS, your local council and the Home Office yourself. You may come up against stiff opposition, and find yourself embroiled in endless legal wrangles.

Further information on inter-country adoption is available from the Home Office, Immigration and Nationality Department, Lunar House, Croydon, Surrey CR9 2BY.

Who can adopt?

If you are thinking of adopting a child with special needs (i.e. from one of the categories mentioned above), you will find that there are no specific upper age limits and that anyone can apply to adopt. Families with children, childless couples, divorced and single people can – and do – all become adoptive parents. You must be over 21 years old, however, and provide what social workers consider to be a suitable, stable environment for a child to grow up in. If you are a couple, and wish to adopt jointly, you must be married to each other.

If you are very keen to adopt a *baby*, you will find that age limits are in force. These vary from area to area, but are between 32 and 40 years. The reason for these age limits is that agencies want to place babies and young children with parents who are young enough to provide a stable home for them right through their childhood and adolescence, and who will be alive and active into the child's adulthood.

If you are voluntarily childless and are choosing adoption in preference to having your own birth-children, you may find yourself up against a brick wall of suspicion. Social workers will ask searching questions about why you want to adopt, and may be worried that you will later change your mind and have birth-children, relegating your adopted child (or children) to a 'second class' role in the family. If one of you has been sterilized, this may reduce the opposition; but some authorities may turn you down. If this happens, 'shopping around' is the only option.

You will also find that adoption agencies are very keen on placing children with parents of the same racial background, as this is believed to be very beneficial to the child. In all matters, the agencies are putting the needs of the child first.

The adoption process

In order to adopt, you must first apply to your local authority, or to a voluntary adoption agency. There are almost 200 of these in this country, and these are listed, region by region, at the end of this chapter. Remember that you must apply to an agency which deals with your part of the country. Some agencies are specialized and have their own requirements for prospective parents (e.g. religious agencies).

An alternative is to apply to the Exchange service run by the British Agencies for Adoption and Fostering (BAAF). This is a service which deals only with children with special needs who are looking for a permanent family. BAAF will supply you with an application form which will help them to put you in touch with a suitable agency (their address is at the end of this chapter). If your application is accepted, your social worker will tell the Exchange about you.

'Be My Parent' is a scheme run by BAAF to bring children who need homes into contact with people interested in adopting them. These children have special needs. Originally the scheme took the form of a loose-leaf book containing the photographs and profiles of hundreds of children looking for homes. But this proved rather unwieldy; so in October 1990 BAAF launched its new tabloid newspaper – *Be My Parent* – which is mailed directly to people who are interested in adopting or fostering one or more children with special needs.

The outer pages (which are widely available in doctors' surgeries, libraries, adoption agencies etc.) contain general information about adoption and fostering, together with profiles of some of the people who have benefitted from the scheme. The inner pages (available by subscription only) contain the profiles of children who are looking for homes.

You can subscribe to *Be My Parent* by writing direct to BAAF (address given at the end of this chapter), and enclosing a cheque or postal order for £5, made payable to BAAF. The newspaper will be sent directly to your home.

Once you have applied for approval, a social worker will make an appointment to visit you at home for an informal discussion, and you will be encouraged to ask questions. If you are still interested, you then complete a formal application form. You will be asked for the names of two referees, who know you well and can comment on your experience/ability with children.

You will also have to undergo a medical examination by your GP to check that you are in good health, and to find out if there is any medical condition which might, in the future, affect your ability to look after a child. The agency will also contact the police to find out if you have any convictions which would make you unsuitable as an adoptive parent. Many minor offences, such as speeding, would probably not affect your application, but it is advisable to be completely honest with your social worker.

The social worker will then make several home visits, to find out as much as possible about you and your family, and how a new child or children would fit in. Quite a lot of personal information will need to be divulged at this stage.

Most agencies will ask you to take part in group meetings and/or training sessions with other prospective families. These are led by social workers and experienced adoptive parents. You should be given plenty of guidance about how to deal with difficult situations and with children with special needs and problems.

A second social worker will probably visit you to provide a 'second opinion'. Your application will then go before the Adoption Panel, which makes the final decision.

WHO MAKES A GOOD ADOPTIVE PARENT?

Of course, it's all very well thinking out the practicalities: Will I be accepted? Can I afford to be a parent? and so on, but what about the biggest question of all? What about the question of whether or not you will make a good adoptive parent?

If you have fertility problems and have always wanted children, adoption may seem like the last resort, your only chance to have a child of your 'own'. But adopting a child is not exactly the same as giving birth to one. It isn't a substitute for childbirth, and may not always be the right option in cases of infertility. To quote Clare Baxter, herself an adoptive parent:

> Adoption is more like getting married than having your own baby. You make that commitment and you do grow to love them, but you don't always feel that love, and it's the commitment that sees you through.

As we saw in Chapter 1, not everyone is happy about welcoming in a child who has two different natural parents; and some men feel uncomfortable about fathering a child to whom they have no genetic link. Women may feel that adopting a child just 'isn't the same' as giving birth to the child of a joyous sexual and spiritual union.

And it's true: adopting a child *may not* fulfil the desperate need which some women feel to procreate, to bring forth life from their own bodies. Nor will it satisfy the need of a man to pass on his genetic inheritance. It does, however, allow loving individuals and couples to share their love and their home with another human being, to share in its growth and development, and to pass on their wisdom and knowledge about life. If you want to adopt, you have to have a genuine and enduring love of children – *all* children – not just the child of your own flesh.

From time to time, an individual or couple may feel that they do not wish to give birth to their own children, but they do want to share their lives with one or more children. Sometimes this is because of environmental or other ideological considerations (adoption does not add to the world's population total, and offers a home to a child in need); but at other times the reasons are more deeply personal, and harder to express. Adoption and fostering also offer hope of parenthood to gay and lesbian people who do not feel able to have birth-children. Opposition to lesbian and gay adoption is well-known, and social workers are also often suspicious of the fertile couple who choose not to have their own children yet wish to adopt; but successful adoptions can and do take place. You just have to be persistent and genuine.

Pamela Stevenson, of the Children's Society, believes that it is important for adoptive parents to be:

> ... child-orientated, with stickability and a sense of humour.

Tony Skinner, Director of Childlink, believes it is vital that prospective parents should enjoy participating in children's lives and be prepared to stand by them through thick and thin:

> Being able to stick bizarre situations and being able to laugh and cry with children – not just wanting to fulfil your own adult dreams.

Bridgit O'Mara, of Lewisham Home Finders, stresses that adoptive parents must not expect a child's problems to be sorted out overnight. They must be patient, and she looks for people who:

> ... can take a long-term view and don't expect everything to be sorted out in a year's time. Also, I look for people who are relaxed and feel OK about themselves – people who won't feel embarrassed when a child misbehaves in public.

What is perhaps most important is that adoptive parents must be prepared to adapt their lives to fit in with the child, and not merely expect the child to fit in with the status quo. They must make space and time for the child, and make sure that – if for example they are out at work all day – they have made adequate arrangements for the child to be cared for in their absence.

Adopting a child can be extremely rewarding, but it is also stressful and a real challenge: so you need to be absolutely sure that you are doing the right thing – for you and for the child.

THE EXPERIENCE OF ADOPTION

Hannah and Simon live in London and have two adopted children – Katie (3 years) and Sarah (6 months). Hannah is American, and works as a literary agent. When they met, Hannah and Simon knew that they would not be able to have children. They thought about adoption for a long time before deciding to go ahead with their application. Katie was adopted in Britain, through Childlink, but the family had such difficulty in finding a second child to adopt in Britain that they decided to go overseas, and Sarah was adopted in the United States.

Hannah and Simon decided that they wanted to adopt a young baby, as Hannah wished to continue working.

> I don't intend to give up my career, and if you choose to adopt a toddler who's been through several foster placements, I think it's only fair that you must be there 100 per cent of the time. I wouldn't have felt comfortable. With a baby, she's used to my working. She knows that Mummy works. It's not a strange thing.

Hannah found significant differences between the British and American adoption processes:

> In America, anybody can adopt. But in America, it is a very hands-on system, and you have to be a person who can take a lot of pressure and difficult situations, and use bureaucracy and push your way through the system. The agency only comes into play when you have made an arrangement with a mother. You contact a lawyer, who leads you through a system of placing newspaper ads. Then the agency comes into play. Most of the time, you meet the mother, and maybe

even the mother and father. It's not just single mothers. We had three mothers offering us their babies.

With Childlink, once they have accepted you, you are told to 'go away, and we'll call you'. Six or eight months later, we got a call saying there's a baby, pick her up on Monday. In some ways, it's easier. You are just suddenly handed the baby. But you may wait for years. In America, you have to be prepared to spend a minimum of £10 000. You have to be assessed here by an American certified social worker, who is paid by the hour.

One of the most difficult parts of the adoption process, in any country, is the assessment, as Hannah testifies:

Assessment is intrusive, definitely, because I found especially with the British system that they spent an enormous amount of time trying to find out how I felt about being infertile. We were very lucky because we met knowing I couldn't have children, so it doesn't affect the stability of the marriage. But they are very intrusive about it. It's very difficult to have to speak to strangers again and again about such subjects. And you are always trying to give the right answers. It is a very personal subject that you can't always perform about. There are a lot of very detailed questions about your background. They force you to think about what you are doing, and whether you really want to do it. How will you incorporate children into your family?

Preparation is an important part of the adoption process, especially for parents who, like Hannah, have never had any experience of small children before. Once they had been accepted by Childlink, Hannah and Simon spent a lot of time watching other parents, practising changing nappies and so on, but they were never offered any formal training or lessons in childcare. Hannah was fortunate, because Katie's foster mother had already got her into a stable care routine, and allowed Hannah to spend time watching her care for the baby. Hannah admits more training would have been useful, but adds:

Just being confident that you are going to get through it is half the battle. Some people are better than others, but everyone can manage it if it's what they really want.

In the event, Hannah and Simon found themselves 'thrown in at the deep end' of parenthood, as they had only four days' notice with the British adoption, and even with the American adoption they were worried that it might fall through:

> You have to be incredibly flexible. You just don't know when it's going to happen. You can't count on it until it's with you, which is a drawback. You are on tenterhooks for ages. The mother can always change her mind. The shock of having a baby is pretty dramatic – it changes any sort of normal life for you as a couple.

Flexibility doesn't just mean the ability to adapt in a practical way. It also means a willingness to accept and love any child you are given:

> When they call and say there's a child, you must be able to accommodate it. You have to be prepared to love and accept what you get. You have no way of knowing. You really do have to go into it thinking all children are equal and lovable. And they're not going to be like you – any more than natural children would be. And they're not going to be like each other, either. If we do our jobs all right, we hope we will be insured against rejection later in life, but you never know.

Hannah's advice to would-be adoptive parents is to gain as much experience of children as possible, to find out if you really like them and want to be a parent. And she stresses that it's no use simply being with children when they're well-behaved. To gain a fair impression of them, you need to:

> ... go there at six o'clock, when they're being hellish, and find out what it's like. You have to like children in all their phases.

Becoming a parent has not prevented Hannah from continuing to work, but it has slowed down her career development. She also warns prospective adopters that they are embarking upon a long and arduous process:

> Adopting is very, very difficult. You have to be prepared to wait for a terribly long time, and in the end you may not be

successful. And the stress of going through the process is one factor you have to take into account. It is terribly stressful, and you have to have a supportive partner.

However, she has no regrets at all about adopting Katie and Sarah:

> It's the most wonderful thing in the world, and I'm so glad that my husband really said to me 'you must do it, because you would be a great mother', and that I really had the courage to say that I would go for it. I would have lost something that I wouldn't have understood if I hadn't gone for it. There's no such thing as perfect parents. Children are immensely adaptable. As long as you love the children, that's really all that counts.

CHOOSING ADOPTION

Clare and Bill could have had their own birth-children, but they chose instead to adopt a six-year-old girl, Katie. That was three years ago. Clare explains their decision:

> Adoption was always a possible option for me. I was very unhappy when I was a teenager. My sister had lots of problems and was in a psychiatric hospital. I felt I couldn't take on the responsibility of bringing a child into the world. It was a big factor. Environmental considerations also came into my decision.
>
> I did go through a phase of wanting a baby when I was in my early 20s, because I selfishly wanted someone to love me, but then I went off the idea, and when I met Bill I said I didn't want children and he ought to consider the fact. He said he wasn't bothered.
>
> A couple of years later *he* also went through a phase of wanting a baby, but I still didn't. We talked about adoption, and the idea grew over the years. We always thought it might be something we'd want to do, but the time was never quite right.

Clare and Bill talked more seriously about adoption:

> We both wanted a child and felt we could offer love, stability and commitment. Bill felt less strongly than me to begin with ... but after thinking about it he was very happy about

adopting. You have both got to be in agreement over it. We felt 'there are all these children that desperately need homes', and didn't particularly want our own baby. We felt we should adopt an older child, not a baby. We didn't feel that the child had to be our own flesh and blood, that we needed to reproduce ourselves or anything.

One day, they decided that the time finally was right, and had a chat with Clare's sister's boyfriend, who was a social worker. He said that adoption might be a problem, as they could have their own children: they'd need to be very clear in their minds about why they wanted to adopt.

In the event, trying to adopt proved to be a long and involved process. First of all, they approached their local authority and attended an initial meeting. After six months they had still heard nothing, and on ringing up, Clare discovered that they had lost all record of them! A social worker eventually called, but nothing came of it. The department was in such chaos that all adoption work had ground to a halt.

In the meantime they had joined the information service PPIAS, who recommended another London authority, they found out that the borough also had a child on its books who might be suitable for them. They went through the nine-month assessment period and took a preparation course, but when their application went forward to the panel there was opposition from other social workers. Eventually they were approved, but once more nothing came of their application.

After Clare and Bill had contacted another twenty local authorities, they finally saw Katie in the PPIAS newsletter. Once again they applied, and were accepted onto a preparatory course. Despite their having already been approved by one local authority, they had to go through the whole assessment procedure again. Their social worker managed to get their application approved, and Katie finally came to live with them in the summer of 1989.

At the age of six, Katie had been in care for three years, and was unhappy about leaving her foster home. She and her brothers and sisters (who had been placed elsewhere) had all been subjected to sexual abuse, and Katie took a long time to settle in, as Clare recalls:

> She had had about seven foster homes and an adoptive placement breakdown, so it was very difficult and it took her months to accept me. She was very very hostile and aggressive. She kept attacking me all the time. In fact, that was why the other adoptive placement had broken down. She just seemed to change almost overnight after about four months. She suddenly decided that she could trust me enough to allow herself to love me and in fact became almost too much the other way. She was always very jealous of my relationship with Bill, and did her utmost to come between us – it's amazing how manipulative children can be!

Three years on, Katie is fully integrated into the family, and Clare and Bill are very happy that they decided to adopt her. They are now thinking of adopting a second child. But they are both quick to stress that adopting an older child is not like having a birth-child, and that it has its own problems:

> It's not a substitute for having your own children. It is different. It's not the same, but it can be just as rewarding. There's still a tendency for some people to think that if you give children a loving home, they will settle down and get over everything that's happened to them, but you can't just wipe out years of abuse and neglect. They still have problems, and you have to accept that and help them come to terms with them. Even if you adopt a baby, unless you get it straight from the hospital at a few days old, you should be prepared for the fact that it may have experienced traumas that will affect its adjustment.

It took Clare and Bill a long time to achieve their ambition of adopting a child, and Clare believes that it was only their obstinacy that saw them through:

> You must be absolutely determined and bloody-minded about it, and then you'll get there in the end. But you have got to be prepared to fight. It is very hard because you feel so vulnerable. You are in the hands of the social workers and you don't want to say the wrong thing. You feel you want to be yourself, but then you worry that you have been too honest and put your foot in it. The big problem is that they worry that you will then go ahead and have your own children after the adoption. You can't prove that you won't,

and can only hope that you can get them to trust you. Bill offered to have a vasectomy but eventually they said there was no need.

PITFALLS OF THE ADOPTION PROCESS

As we have seen, getting through the adoption process can be quite a minefield. If you are genuinely committed to bringing up a child, your determination should see you through in the end. But many people are turned down at the first hurdle – the home assessment – because the social workers identify unresolved problems. These may include:

- unresolved grief about infertility: the child could be made to feel that it was inferior to the unborn birth-children which the couple were unable to have
- an unstable home environment (e.g. a poor relationship between husband and wife)
- in the case of couples who are not infertile an unsatisfactory explanation of why adoption is preferred to having birth-children
- unwillingness to accept any child other than a newborn baby.

Fostering

Contrary to popular belief, fostering *isn't* a back door to adoption. To quote a BAAF publication:

> Fostering is looking after someone else's child in your home as if it were a member of your family. Usually the child will return to his or her own family after a short while, perhaps within a few weeks or months – or s/he may stay for some years. Fostering isn't the back door to adoption. You have to get used to seeing a child leaving your home, a child you've grown to love.

Fostering placements can range from the very short term (looking after a child for a few days whilst his/her parent is in hospital, for example) to arrangements which last for years. In a few cases, long-term fostering may lead to adoption, but this is very much the exception.

Part of the job of a foster parent is to prepare a child for his or her next move – either back home, or into a permanent, adoptive home. You may also have to work with the child's natural parent or parents, who usually visit their child while in your care. This means that you will be involved in easing the traumas of uncertainty and separation for both the child and his/her parents – and all the time trying yourself to come to terms with your growing affection for a child who will almost certainly be leaving you.

On the positive side, fostering can be extremely rewarding; for it can bring a great sense of achievement when the child who came to you anxious and upset leaves much more cheerful and confident.

Foster parents receive an allowance from the local authority, to cover costs, and there are additional allowances if the child has disabilities.

You may choose to specialize – in small babies, for example, or in disturbed or delinquent teenagers, in which case you will receive extra training. In any event, you will receive plenty of advice and support from your social worker.

If you are interested in becoming a foster parent, you should first contact the fostering officer at your local authority, who will provide more information and arrange for a social worker to call on you for a general discussion.

For further information, contact the National Foster Care Association (address at the end of the book), who exist to encourage a high standard of foster care, and produce a quarterly magazine.

Lesbian and gay parenting

Being single does not necessarily pose a barrier to becoming an adoptive or foster parent. But being lesbian or gay is a rather different story.

The question of whether lesbian and gay people can make good parents is a highly controversial one, and many people see homosexual households as a corrupting influence upon children. Richard Whitfield, Emeritus Professor of Education at Aston University and Chairman of the National Family Trust, is in no doubt about the undesirability of having homosexual parents:

> For children to stand the best chance of thriving in our culture

they need, ideally, to experience the unconditional love of a mother and a father who are committed both to the child and to each other.

Professor Richard Whitfield writing in *Community Care* magazine

Interestingly, research projects have so far failed to detect any harmful effects to children from living in a lesbian or gay household. An article in the *British Medical Journal* in 1991 concluded that children in homosexual households: '. . . did not differ in terms of gender identity, sex role behaviour, sexual orientation, emotions, behaviour, and relationships' from children in heterosexual households. Nor did they appear to have been bullied or teased by other children at school; and sexual abusers were just as likely to be heterosexual as homosexual ('Homosexuality and parenthood', Michael B. King and Pat Pattison, *BMJ*, Vol 303, 3 August 1991).

Nicolas Rea (Baron Rea) is a father of five and staunch advocate of the rights of lesbians to become parents. His mother was a lesbian, and he was brought up 'with unusual love' in a household which included her long-time lover. He believes that:

A well adjusted, properly motivated lesbian couple could make an excellent home for children, as long as the children are allowed to develop their own sexual orientation.

'Brought up with unusual love', *The Times*, 25 February 1991

Despite the lack of damning evidence, many lesbian mothers have lost their children in court custody battles, and it is rare indeed for a homosexual father to gain custody of his child.

In the face of all this hostility, some lesbian women are opting for single parenthood, using artificial insemination (a practice which has become rather less popular since the AIDs epidemic, as homosexual men were often used as donors). A much larger number of lesbian women and gay men are looking to adoption and fostering to provide them with the experience of parenthood. But the path is not a smooth one in a society which believes that children need both a father and a mother, and it requires great determination to gain acceptance – as the following two case-studies show.

Don Smart and John Elderton are foster parents, and have been together for more than 20 years. For the last 11 years, they have been caring for Danny, a Down's syndrome boy who is now 17. Danny's mother knew them and was happy about the arrangement from the start, but Oxfordshire county council was not so sure. They did not file an objection to this private arrangement, but (according to Don) made it clear that they were unhappy. The reason for their hostility is not difficult to identify: Don and John are an openly homosexual couple.

Don and John applied for formal approval as foster parents, as they wanted to take in other children; but the social services department told them that they would only be assessed if a suitable child was found. So far, they have not found one . . .

Pat Romans and Judith Weekes also live in Oxfordshire. They fostered large numbers of difficult and disturbed children between 1974 and 1984, but it was not until 1984 that they decided to tell the social services department about their sexuality. They are now trying to persuade other lesbian and gay carers to come out, because:

> By hiding it, you open the children to blackmail.
> 'Can gay couples be good parents?', *The Independent on Sunday*, 10 March 1991

But the dilemma faced by lesbian and gay people is that if they are up-front about their sexuality, they face a very high chance of rejection.

Fiona is a member of LAGFAN – the Lesbian and Gay Fostering and Adoption Network – a small support group which meets on a monthly basis at London Friends. She explains the group's work:

> We talk about our progress in the fostering/adoption system, how we are feeling, and do a certain amount of campaigning work. We are in touch with a wider network across the country. We are also in touch with BAAF and NFCA, and they are very supportive. We are hoping to write some general leaflets with these two organisations, and we recently held a conference at which we had 30–35 people from various parts of the country.

Some of the group's members have been successful in fostering or adopting children: for example, a gay couple and a lesbian are doing respite care, one gay male couple are fostering, and one lesbian couple fostering with a view to adoption. However, the majority of members are still waiting, hoping and trying:

> A lot of people just feel that the whole situation is impossible, but there are some who have been fostering for years and years. Some weren't out at first, but have come out and been accepted because it's obvious they're doing a good job.
>
> A number of us have been approved by Social Services but then there's no child or children available because the social workers whose clients they are will not regard a lesbian or gay home as the best possible option. There seems to be a bit of an exception with sexually abused girls and teenagers who have already decided they are lesbian or gay. But it is very much up to individual social workers to take us up and sell us, as it were. You are definitely screened more closely.

Fiona's advice to lesbian and gay individuals and couples considering fostering or adoption is:

- it is difficult to gain acceptance, but it may be easier to foster than to adopt
- it may be easier to gain acceptance if you are lesbians willing to foster sexually abused girls, or if you want a child with a disability. Men seem to be more acceptable for adolescents
- 'feel the waters' in areas that are fairly local to you. Authorities have vastly differing policies, and whereas some are very hostile, others do not question you about your sexuality, and some are very positive
- be prepared for ignorance: you may be asked some very strange questions, even if social workers are supportive. People will make a lot of assumptions about you
- be prepared for very close screening.

Weighing up the pros and cons

Adoption and fostering are not direct substitutes for biological parenting, and you need to consider very carefully the reasons why you want to adopt or foster a child.

- Why do you want to adopt/foster a child?
- Would it matter to you, or to your partner, that the child you were looking after was not biologically your own?
- How would you feel about giving back a child you had fostered to his or her natural parents?
- How would you feel if your adopted son or daughter decided to get in touch with his or her natural parents? (Would you feel cheated or betrayed?)
- Would you be happy to explain to your son or daughter that he or she was adopted?
- If you adopted a child and later gave birth to one of your own, would you feel any differently towards your adopted child?

6
Coping with Other People's Attitudes

It's easy to think that making your choice is the hardest part, and that once the choice is made things will get easier. This isn't necessarily so, because – as well as making your own adjustments – you have the rest of the world and its opinions to contend with. Having children may bring many changes and problems, but it certainly removes many social barriers and creates an atmosphere of approval: people are happy with you. Deciding not to have children, by contrast, can be traumatic. *You* may have some difficulty in coming to terms with your decision, but other people may find it downright incomprehensible. As we have seen, other people's attitudes towards the childless or child-free can range from cloying sympathy to open antagonism: surprisingly few people seem able to cope easily with the concept of people who are content to live their lives without children. But present your decision to the world in the right way, and other people can help you to create a new and positive outlook on life.

This chapter is about deciding how to present your child-free state to other people, and how to help other people to help you, by understanding your point of view and respecting your decisions and wishes.

Why other people's attitudes seem to matter

None of us lives life in a vacuum. We're all only too aware of the impact other people's opinions and observations have on the way we feel about ourselves. We may say 'It's all water off a duck's back', but if we're honest, we have to admit that it hurts when people are insensitive or critical. And most of us feel the need to live up to certain norms which society has tacitly agreed.

THE CRITICAL EYE
People who do not conform to society's norms are liable to be regarded as eccentric or weird; and society doesn't have a particularly high tolerance level for individuality. So, people who

are very large, or who have a different sexual orientation, or who live an itinerant life, or who wear 'outlandish' clothes, or who are in any way extra-ordinary are liable to come in for some pretty scathing criticism. Although this criticism may be veiled ('I'm only saying this for your own good, dear . . .'), it is nevertheless there: 'I'm criticizing you because you're different'.

Objectively, other people's views of what we do don't really matter. They only matter because most of us feel uncomfortable with disapproval. One way to combat this feeling is to marshal your arguments in advance, so that when someone makes an oblique remark or a cutting comment, you have a reply ready. What matters is being secure in your own point of view, sure of what you feel and the direction which you have chosen for your life. And it is *your* life, no one else's; no one else has the right to make you feel bad about yourself. And those who really care about you won't try.

MISPLACED SYMPATHY

When we are suffering, sympathy can be a great comfort: it's nice to know that there is someone else out there, sharing our sorrows and empathizing with our pain; it feels good to reach out to someone and feel warmth and understanding. But the trouble with sympathy is to gauge it correctly. Sometimes sympathy isn't the most appropriate response to a situation, and – if taken to extremes – can even do more harm than good. For example, the child-free couple who have decided that their relationship is strong and self-sufficient without children may be faced with a barrage of well-meaning but misplaced sympathy from everyone they meet. Yet it is important to recognize that the sentiment is in fact insulting because it patronizes and emasculates a very conscientious serious stance.

But it can be a tough job announcing your decision to the world every time someone makes elliptical remarks about children. Even if you try to be upfront about it, people may not always understand what you are saying. If they like you, they may think: 'No one so pleasant and kind and sociable could be childless by choice', and assume that you are just being brave. They have been brought up to think that people who don't have children are egoistic, but they don't want to believe that you are, because you are their friend. If people don't like you to start off with, they will probably use your child-free state as an excuse to like you even less.

Why tell anyone?

By now, you may be wondering why you should make a point of telling anyone at all about your childless or child-free state. It's your life. What's more, it's a very private and sensitive topic. Why should the world and his wife have to know all your innermost thoughts and secrets?

The answer is, of course, that they don't. It's your decision. But silence has its own pressures. People will continue to watch, listen, wait for that first sign of an impending pregnancy. Take the example of the farmer's wife who complained bitterly that everyone in her village was watching and waiting for her to become pregnant, whilst she had in fact quietly but determinedly decided to concentrate on taking a university degree! Or the Greek Cypriot woman whose mother prevailed upon her to lie to the local priest and tell him that she would have children 'in time', because she feared a scene which would bring disgrace upon the entire family. And of course there are lots of couples with fertility problems who avoid talking about the subject at all, because they find it so distressing.

If you do decide to 'go public', you can expect to be greeted with initial surprise or shock, possibly followed by arguments and hostility. Frustrated grandparents may deal with the situation by sulking, which can be just as difficult to deal with. But at least you will have brought out into the open the feelings which you have carried within you for so long. If you have opted for childlessness because of infertility or medical problems, you will have an opportunity to explain to people how you feel, and the factors which helped you to make your decision. If you have decided to be child-free, the process of explanation may be painful – but you are giving yourself a chance to escape, once and for all, from the endless pressures and probing questions.

When enough is enough

Perhaps you initially intended to have children, but found that there was a problem which would make parenthood impossible or morally unacceptable for you.

If you wanted children, but have decided on a child-free lifestyle because of medical or fertility problems, you will probably find that other people's reactions are divided between awkwardness, sympathy and puzzlement. Some people will accept, without question, that what you are doing is the best way to break free of the cycle of hope and despair; some will feel embarrassed and awkward, and not know what to say to you; others won't understand why you aren't persevering: for them any chance of a child – no matter how small – has to be worth taking, even if at the end there is nothing but grief and emptiness. They may find it difficult to see that the grief of saying 'enough' is as nothing compared to the grief of years wasted on treatments which have produced – not a child – only pain and a sense of deep failure.

In difficult cases like these, you have to remember that you cannot force someone to share your opinion of what you have done and decided. At best, you may only be able to make them admit that you have a right to do and say what you feel is best for you and your partner. No one has a right to browbeat or blackmail you into parenthood.

If your family and friends know that you have been thinking of starting a family, or that you have been undergoing fertility treatments, you will need to let them know about your change of heart. You are going to need support over the coming months and years, to help you come to terms with the implications of your decision. Telling your family and close friends about what you have decided, and why, helps to make your decision final, and helps those who are close to you to understand your motivation.

If you have never spoken to anyone about your desire for children, now is your chance to end the uncertainty, the wonderings, the whisperings.

What should you say, and how should you say it?

Once you have decided on the course of action you are going to take, you and your partner need to get together and decide exactly what you are going to tell people. Are you going to hold a family get-together and tell everyone at once? Are you going to tell individual friends and relatives that you have decided not to pursue your quest for parenthood any further? And exactly what are you going to tell them, and why?

You will need to marshall your arguments very carefully, and accept that there will be people who simply cannot – or simply don't want to – understand your point of view. People who perhaps think that you are acting out of a materialistic desire to have a better standard of living; or simply those who think that they know what's best for you (and that if you are allowed to pursue this course of action, you will end up regretting it bitterly). They therefore keep working away at you, in the hope that you will give in and have a child.

The best thing to do may be to tell the truth, however unpopular it may prove. If you don't like children, why not say so? If you feel you don't have what it takes to be a parent, far better to admit it than to have children to please other people!

The process of announcing your decision needs sensitive handling. If your decision is the result of genetic counselling, it is likely that your family will already have some understanding of the medical problems which you have been battling against. There may be family members who suffer from the disorder, and it is important that you stress how much you value and care about them, even though you have decided not to bring any children into the world yourself. If your family have ideological or religious beliefs which forbid birth control, you will also need to consider carefully how you put your message across.

What you say, and the way in which you put across your message, will to a large extent determine other people's responses. If you burst into tears and show great distress, no amount of insistence on your part is going to convince those around you that you regard childless living in a positive light. Very likely, the response will be an outpouring of sympathy which may or may not make you feel better.

This is not to say that you should make light of what is obviously going to be a dreadfully upsetting experience for all concerned. Apart from your own grief, you are bound to be aware of the ways in which your own childlessness affects other people around you. Perhaps you are an only child, and your parents were looking forward to the arrival of their first grandchild? There are all sorts of psychological undercurrents like this, and it can be hard not to lose sight of your own needs.

If you are in a stable relationship, try to emphasize this fact and show that you are united in love and mutual support; that neither of you 'blames' the other for what has happened; that your decision is a joint one, and not just a question of there being something 'wrong' with one of the two partners. Make sure that you show your solidarity and affection for one another, too. You will need each other's love and support more than ever at this difficult time.

Dealing with people's reactions

Many people end up telling lies to get people off their back and deflect the inevitable disapproval. It's very tempting, when asked: 'When are you going to have kids?', to reply 'Oh, in a year or two's time, maybe', or something along those lines. It's much tougher to come out with the truth: 'We've never felt the need for children, so we won't be having any' – a bold statement, but honest, which almost always results in a shocked or negative reaction.

Obviously, it is up to you whether you decide to be open about your decision. Though remember, it took great courage to make your choice in the first place. If you have chosen against parenthood, the chances are that you have the courage and the conviction necessary to be truly honest with your family and friends. But you will still need to prepare yourself for a bumpy ride. You'll probably have to repeat your message many times before you are truly believed, and there may be family members who never quite come to terms with your life choices (but *that*, of course, can happen *whatever* you do!). You may be able to smooth the way a little, by confiding in a friend or relative whom you and your family both trust, and who can act as an intermediary, helping to put forward your point of view and backing you up when things get tough.

You need to sit down with each of the people you tell and tell them, honestly, what you feel. You will need to stress that your decision is a positive one (you could have risked having a child, or persevered with treatment, but you chose to call a halt). Show that you have taken your decision together because you want to be in control of your lives from now on. You have accepted your situation, and hope that they will accept it, too. Explain, also, what support you think they could offer you; what it is you want from them.

It is best not to allow yourselves to be drawn into family arguments nor to let family members make comparisons. If you've done your homework and been honest with yourselves, then the courage of your convictions fronted by a gentle but firm assertive stance should see you through.

Anticipating some questions – and reactions – may help you, and you and your partner could act out ('role play') different family members and their likely responses as part of your preparation. Also ask your friends and relatives what they would like to know. By giving them the information you want them to have, you will be helping them to help you. There are bound to be questions like the following, which they may be just too afraid to ask:

- would it upset you if I talked about my own children?
- would you prefer it if I didn't bring my children when I come to visit you; or would you like to spend more time with them, so that you can develop a closer relationship with them?

So, take the initiative.

Talking about child-free living

Sabine is German and a member of BON. She and her boyfriend have never wanted children, and they are very open about their decision not to become parents:

> I do find it very hard sometimes to bring across to people that it is not my life's ambition to walk down the aisle and raise kids. They often can't believe or accept that we are happy. . . . The majority of people seem to think that when a couple don't want kids it must be because of career reasons. This is not true in our case. . . . Another group of people seem to think that the decision not to have kids arises out of a lack of responsibility or even laziness. Again this is absolutely wrong. . . . Why is it so difficult for most people to understand that someone simply doesn't want kids? Why does it have to be for reasons like a career, or travel plans, or whatever? They make it sound like 'one is born to reproduce', and if they don't feel the need there must be something wrong. Why can't it be seen as a choice of how somebody wants to live?

ASSERTING YOUR RIGHTS AND WISHES

Being assertive means asserting your right to express your wishes and opinions, and to have them taken into account and respected by those around you. In turn, you make an effort to listen to and respect their points of view.

Self-assertion means not letting other people walk all over you. But it doesn't mean shouting at people and walking all over them! It means putting your message across, quietly and with control; and then listening to the counter-arguments. You may have to repeat the message again and again, but if you are truly assertive you will not be ignored. Never raise your voice or lose your temper. You can be angry and assertive, but shouting abuse is simply another way of losing control. By keeping your cool, you maintain control of the situation and cannot be browbeaten or wrongfooted.

If you have 'difficult' relatives, it's only by being assertive that you will, ultimately, get your message across. If you have difficulty in putting across your views, why not take an assertiveness course? Most local colleges and adult institutes run short courses aimed at helping you to state your point of view calmly and with concern for the other person's perspective. These courses can be very valuable for anyone who is timid and often browbeaten by people with strong personalities, or for anyone who has a quick temper and tends to behave aggressively. A list of useful books and addresses is given at the end of this book.

Here are some points to think about if you anticipate having difficulty in getting your message across:

- having children is not compulsory (nor is liking them)
- the world is tragically full of unhappy children whose parents didn't really want them
- you aren't hard and insensitive, just because you've decided not to have children. You have other things to offer your families and the world
- choosing not to have children is not selfish. In fact the 'selfish' argument is a non-sequitur
- it would be very foolish – and selfish – to comply with the wishes of your families and friends; and it is foolish and selfish of them to pressurize you in any way
- you may be someone's child, but you are adults now, capable of and needing to make responsible decisions, for yourselves.

7
The Rest of Your Life

Perhaps you wanted children, but decided that the emotional or medical costs were too high. Perhaps you are happy to be child-free at the moment but, at some time in the future, you may think about fostering or adoption. Or perhaps you have quite simply never wanted children at all. Life is full of 'perhapses' and 'maybes'. Whatever is – or isn't – going to happen to you in the future, you have a life here and now; and you owe it to yourself to spend time and effort making that life worth living. Just because you don't have children, that doesn't mean that your life should lack fulfilment. On the contrary, without the financial and emotional ties that children bring, you are far freer to fulfil yourself in any of a thousand different ways.

You have an important relationship with your partner, too; and you need to be sure that you both understand the implications of your future lives together. From now on, your lives will just be about the two of you and the social circle you create around you. From time to time, a situation will arise, something will be said or you read or see some scenario or image which challenges you and threatens to undermine the ground you have covered, your choice, and new life. Try not to look back and don't let regret take hold. Instead see and use such events as an opportunity for reappraisal, for confirmation; as a chance to strengthen your conviction and to consolidate your choice and new-found freedom.

Coming to terms with childlessness

If you have made the decision not to continue trying for a child, now is the time to begin reconstructing and recreating your lives according to a new model. Instead of being a couple waiting to start a family, you will now become a self-contained family unit of two people who care about each other and the world and who want to live together and share good and bad times.

Already you will have been through some pretty powerful rollercoaster emotions together, sharing the moments of hope and the long, dark times when hope seemed very far away. You have survived and – most important of all now – you have made a decision about your future. You now need to work together to ensure that your relationship becomes even stronger.

It is important to realize that your choice is more than a resignation, more than an acceptance of loss; it is also a freedom. When you finally turn your back on what is past, realize that you have set yourselves free, free to begin again, free to fulfil yourselves and to give in other, equally valuable, ways.

Child-free living

If you have made a positive choice not to have children, there is still work to be done in terms of strengthening your relationship, acknowledging the 'loss' aspect of your choice, and making the most of the new freedom your choice will bring. And not everyone who makes the decision to remain childless does so in an atmosphere of serene certainty. There will still be doubts and your convictions will be tested.

If you and your partner have worked your way through this book, and through the questions in Chapter 4, you will have reached the decision which feels right for you. If you have any lingering doubts then it may be a good idea to wait a while and then repeat the exercise.

Remember, all choices carry loss and sacrifice: if you have the red dress, you can't have the blue one. Few decisions are truly clear-cut. There may be almost as many pros as there are cons, but at the end of the day you have to choose.

These days, we are accustomed to 'having it all', and to demanding instant, final solutions which will solve all our problems and annihilate our worries at a stroke. We have built up a seething mass of unrealistic aspirations, and this is perhaps why so many marriages end in divorce. We all need to learn to live with the sense of loss which comes from choosing.

A degree of planning – or at least constructive thought – is an important element in achieving a successful child-free lifestyle. It's easy just to drift along, never really thinking much about what you are doing or why. Positive planning helps to give you a sense of direction and purpose in your life. You have made a big, life-changing decision; but nothing will 'happen' overnight. The consequences of your decision and your feelings all need to be worked through – otherwise you can feel depressed, isolated, cut off from the rest of society.

As we have seen in earlier chapters, childless people have to contend with a whole host of prejudices and preconceptions which label them either the victims of cruel misfortune or hard-hearted egoists. Society pities the childless and is often suspicious of the child-free. So it's hardly surprising that many child-free people need to work hard to achieve the sort of life they want, and to gain the support of others.

Building a new life

Choosing childlessness is a challenging option; choosing to be child-free isn't the end of choosing. They are both the beginning of a string of decisions which you will have to make for yourselves over the coming years.

ACCENTUATE THE POSITIVE

One of the first things to do is to make yourself aware of the benefits which accompany your choice. It's a good idea to take a long, hard look at your own life, and make a list of all the positive implications for you of being child-free. Obviously everyone's list will be different, but here's a list prepared by Jennie, a 30-year-old unmarried secretary:

- I have the freedom to travel wherever and whenever I want (socially and on business);
- I can spend my money the way I want it, and I don't have to worry too much about security so I can take chances;
- I can concentrate on doing the best for myself in my career – maybe take time out to study full time for a degree;
- I can enjoy being an aunt to my sister's two little boys;
- I can adopt any lifestyles I choose;
- I have lots of time for my friends, hobbies and pets.

Of course, Jennie's life isn't roses all the way. She has no partner, so she has to find the money for the mortgage out of her own pocket – which is in itself a limitation on her freedom. In order to achieve a balanced view of the future, Jennie also needed to make a list of her worries and fears:

- I'm afraid of being alone, especially when I'm old;

- My job is well paid, and there are opportunities – but it's quite insecure;
- I have to pay the mortgage on my own. What if I get made redundant, or get sick so I can't work?
- I don't want to be stuck on my own in the house – I want to get out and meet people.

Jennie took a look at her lists of benefits and fears, and used them to help her draw up a life plan.

Jennie's life plan
- To get out more socially: I've joined an amateur dramatic club and a rambling club. I don't like dating agencies, besides which I'm not necessarily looking for a husband or lover!
- To work hard at strengthening relationships: not just with my family but with friends I've tended to neglect a bit recently, because of pressure at work.
- To try hard to make the most of my job: and take advantage of all the career and training opportunities on offer. If I don't succeed in getting where I want to be in the next three years, I'm going to think about retraining or maybe taking time out to do a degree.
- To save up for at least one really good holiday a year.
- To pay into a mortgage protection plan: in case I get made redundant.
- To take an active role as an auntie.

The plan lists Jennie's general aims in the short and longer term, and isn't rigid: she can change it at any time, to adapt to changes in her lifestyle and priorities. For example, she might form a permanent relationship, or develop new ambitions.

Try drawing up your own life plan. If you and your partner draw up separate plans to begin with, you can compare them afterwards and identify any possible sources of future conflict which need ironing out.

Enriching your relationship

If you are in a long-term relationship, the prospect of life without children is bound to have an effect upon the ways in which you relate to each other and envisage your future together.

If you have chosen childlessness after discovering fertility or other medical problems, you and your partner may still be suffering the after-effects of disappointment and guilt. In the case of infertility, one partner may be experiencing lingering feelings of guilt about depriving the other partner of a baby. Even when a positive, joint decision has been made in favour of child-free living, the guilt can linger.

Of course, there are no rules about how to conduct a long-term childfree relationship and ensure success. But there are a few points worth bearing in mind:

- be open and honest with each other: lies and secrets can destroy a relationship;
- respect each other's space: being together all the time can be very claustrophobic;
- spend as much time together as you feel comfortable with; but make sure that you have other interests and friendships outside the relationship. Obviously you are both extremely important in one another's eyes, but one partner should not try to live his or her life entirely through the other;
- spend time creating a supportive and interesting network of friends. Research has suggested that the child-free elderly who have a wide social circle actually have more visitors than elderly people with children.

COUNSELLING

In this type of situation, it is extremely important to try to resolve underlying conflicts, and to bring to the surface any negative feelings which may otherwise harm the relationship in the long term. One way of doing this – apart from maintaining an open and honest dialogue with your partner – is to seek specialist counselling. In particular, trained counsellors can help you to stop seeing yourselves as potential parents, and to adjust to your new roles as non-parents and lovers.

Counselling can also help you if you have decided to remain child-free by choice. It can help you to identify ways in which you can grow together, support each other and help each other to achieve direction, self-fulfilment and a sense of personal worth. It can also help you to sort out the best course of action, now that the decision has been made not to have children. Should one of you opt for sterilization? And if so, who? Or do you want to carry on using a more reversible form of contraception (for example if there is any possibility that either of you may change your mind in years to come)?

One problem with childlessness in general is that you may lack a sense of direction, thinking to yourselves: if we're not parents, what are we? What is our function as human beings? And you may end up concentrating on yourselves rather than on each other, and so drift apart.

Counselling is a rigorous process and can sometimes be painful, but it can certainly help to strengthen relationships through openness and honesty and insight.

Where to go for counselling
Relate (formerly the Marriage Guidance Council) counsels anyone who is in a relationships, not just married couples, and can refer clients to a specialist sex therapist where necessary. (A charge is levied for counselling.)

The British Association for Counselling can provide information on a variety of different kinds of counselling (individual, couple counselling, co-counselling etc.). (You will have to pay for counselling.)

The Association for Marriage Enrichment runs courses which encourage married couples to focus on their relationship, and to seek growth and enrichment in their marriages.

Most commonly, the courses take the form of a weekend residential workshop or 'retreat', led by a couple who are experienced in Marriage Enrichment. Groups consist of no more than seven couples, and most work is done privately by each couple. There is no confrontation, and anything shared is confidential to the group. The aim is to help each couple to achieve growth, effective and caring communication, and the ability to use and manage conflict creatively.

Marriage Enrichment was first developed in America in 1962, with the aim of 'making good marriages better'. It reached Britain in 1976, and in 1979 the programme of work came under the auspices of the Church of England's Board of Education, as the Association for Marriage Enrichment (AME).

Although marriage enrichment does have ecclesiastical origins, and some events are organized by the Church, there are many events and courses which have no Church connections and are open to all. Marriage Enrichment is open to couples of all ages, as the Association believes that 'it is never too late to gain new insights into what is potentially the most rewarding of human relationships'.

The AME also run courses in Marriage Preparation, which could be of great value to couples considering making a life together and deciding whether or not to have a family.

When Yvonne and Malcolm married in January 1981, they made a commitment to be honest with each other, even if that honesty was painful. Yvonne had been married before, and both were determined to do everything they could to communicate better and ensure the success of their relationship.

They first heard about Marriage Enrichment (ME) about five years ago, when running a course on Marriage Preparation at their church. They thought no more about it until June 1991, when a pair of leader couples came to lecture on ME as part of a three-year counselling course which Yvonne was taking. Yvonne was very excited by the format, and had no reservations about ME. Malcolm had reservations about the fear of exposure to other couples, but these fears evaporated before they actually attended their first ME weekend, as by then he had also started the three-year counselling course!

Yvonne explains what happens on a ME weekend:

> Marriage Enrichment courses can arouse feelings and emotions which need to be carefully handled. Couples are encouraged to look at and value what is good about their relationship, to remember the love that drew them together, and to confront each other with love. Because of three years of learning listening skills, I did not find it too exhausting, but those couples who had no experience of really listening found it very demanding. Couples should expect to find it painful, funny, loving, frightening.

Malcolm relished the isolation of the ME weekend:

> ME gives space to be alone without any external influence, e.g. the telephone; and the realization that the weekends give a safe environment to reveal innermost thoughts, that I wouldn't be laughed at by others. I didn't go because we had a problem to solve, but with the feeling of 'What can I learn?'

There is no instruction, but it's very much a case of 'here are some skills – they may work for you'. The whole atmosphere is one of positive reinforcement. Both weekends resulted in my feeling closer to Yvonne. As a couple we have grown a lot, take more time to tell each other things and create space for each other in busy lives.

Both Malcolm and Yvonne feel that ME is not the right place to talk over the traumas of infertility, but that the skills taught could help couples to overcome conflicts which arise when one partner wants a child and the other does not:

> It will help the couples to really listen to each other's needs and if necessary help them to realize that they need further help in order for them to reach a satisfactory decision – i.e. seek couple counselling. Resolving conflicts means, first of all, making time and space to discuss the conflict. It's no good trying to resolve any problem when the blood is up; there has to be a measure of calmness and a willingness to listen to each other. We make a time in the diary to discuss conflict, and I've advised other couples to use this method. We discuss the problem, not each other's reactions to it, and then listen to each other's feelings. It's hard and takes practice, but it works eventually and being prepared to listen actually draws couples closer.

As a counsellor, Yvonne has talked with people who are thinking of having children. She advises them to think hard about their motives for wanting children, and – if they decide to go ahead with starting a family – to think well in advance about things like the mother's career, and practicalities such as day-care. The response is often a negative one:

> Whenever I suggest ideas like this to people, some responses are that the spontaneity of creation is removed and it becomes a clinical act. My response is that love means knowing yourself, and your partner, a willingness to learn and listen and to realize that for a child to blossom into a stable, loving, accepting adult, it needs *two* parents who wanted its conception.

Yvonne is in no doubt about what ME has done for her own marriage:

As an individual, I have gained much from ME, in that I now recognize the immense strength in our marriage and that the chance of making another mess as I did in my first marriage is actually slim. I like to make contact with other couples who care about themselves and their marriage, and ME has provided access to such couples. It is not the place for people who are afraid of change, it is a tremendous challenge, but a joy to be part of also.

It takes guts and motivation to take a seat on an ME weekend, but I would recommend it to everyone who can take the challenge.

FRIENDSHIPS

Friends are very important to most people; but they are an especially important part of the lives of the childless and child-free. Interestingly, one research project suggested that, of all elderly people living in residential care homes, it was those who *didn't* have children who received the most visits – perhaps because they had spent a great deal of time building up strong and enduring friendships with people who genuinely cared about them and enjoyed visiting them.

Of course, it takes effort to build up friendships. They have to be worked at and nurtured: friendship is a two-way process. There can often be problems when a resolutely child-free couple find that all their friends have now got children and undergone what appears to be a complete personality transplant. New mothers, in particular, are understandably self-absorbed and wrapped up in the needs and desires and gurgles of their babies. These transformations can be terribly upsetting to the child-free or childless woman who feels that her one-time best friend has been lost to her forever – and friendships between the child-free and those with children certainly require effort. What's more, new friendships can't be forced: they need time and care to grow.

Try the following action points:

- develop interests which bring you into contact with other people as a matter of course: that way, you are bound to meet some with whom you can build good friendships;
- make time for mutual and individual friendships;
- don't give up on your friends just because they have got children and seem to have developed a whole new set of values,

completely different from your own. Make a real effort to keep the friendship going: *they need you*, and things will get easier once the children are a little older.

RELATIVES

As we have seen, relatives can cause problems if they refuse to understand or respect your decision to be child-free. On the plus side, if you are fond if children but either can't have your own or have chosen not to be a parent, taking occasional charge of a relative's offspring can be an interesting and enjoyable experience. It can be great fun being a favourite aunt or uncle: you get to do lots of nice things with the children – and hand them back at the end of the day, when they are tired and fractious! Also, there is a great deal to be gained in terms of mutual affection and the learning and teaching experience.

If you do not have relatives with children, but would like to establish a close relationship with one or more children, another option is to take on the duties and responsibilities of a godparent. Godchildren often confide in their godparents and look to them for advice and support, and this can be a very satisfying experience.

If you have problems with your relatives' attitudes to your childless or child-free state, it should be possible to sort them out through an open and direct approach, as mentioned in the previous chapter.

Self-fulfilment

One of the arguments often advanced in favour of parenthood is that it is the source of a great sense of fulfilment. But many non-parents will tell you that they, too, lead full and satisfying lives; so parenthood is not an infallible recipe for self-fulfilment. And certainly one of the worst ways of trying to find fulfilment is by having children so that you can live your life through them – placing expectations upon them, trying to persuade them to do all the things that you never did, or that you tried and failed to do.

The only sensible way to achieve self-fulfilment is by seeking your own road, ploughing your own furrow. And, even if you are sad and disappointed because nature has thwarted your hopes of being a parent, you must take consolation in the new freedom which being a non-parent will give you – the freedom to find yourself, to develop your interests, to do things which you would probably never be able to do if you had children. Look at the points below, and ask yourself if any of them would fit into your life plan:

- Work: e.g. going self-employed, training for a new job; getting career analysis; going part-time.
- Education and training.
- Voluntary work: e.g. caring work, work with children, charities, youth work, cub scout leader, CAB, Relate, Samaritans, Red Cross, WRVS, conservation groups.
- Hobbies, leisure, travel.
- Saving up to do things you've always wanted to do.

Sterilization

For many people, the natural progression from deciding to be child-free is deciding to be sterilized. After all, if you're not going to have children, why bother with contraception? The most effective, trouble-free and permanent form of contraception is sterilization.

If you are considering sterilization, you will need to be absolutely sure that you are doing the right thing. If you have never had a child, and are in your 20s or 30s, doctors and counsellors will do their best to dissuade you from sterilization – unless there is a good medical reason why you or your partner should not have children. They know from bitter experience that people can and do change their minds. A relationship breaks down, you meet another partner who is really keen on having children, you begin to feel guilty because you cannot give your partner a child . . . and so it goes on. But neither male nor female sterilization should be regarded as reversible: a realistic estimate of the chances of pregnancy after a reversal operation would be no greater than 30 per cent. The time to change your mind is *before* you have the operation done.

That being said, for some child-free people sterilization can be the ideal solution. Mary was 28 when she requested sterilization:

> I'd always known I didn't want kids, and my husband wasn't keen, either. My attitude has always been that I can't face giving up my own life for the sake of a child. There are so many things

I want to do, and if I had a child I couldn't do them. It's my life, and I haven't finished with it yet! I just don't want to live my life through somebody else.

I had a terrible job persuading the consultant that I'd made up my mind and wouldn't change it, but I managed it in the end. Being sterilized was a tremendously liberating experience. I'd always been worried that I might accidentally get pregnant (and I'd have asked for a termination if I had), but now the fear was all gone. People will say I'm selfish, and I don't deny it; but I'm no more selfish than a woman I know, who had a kid as a sort of designer fashion accessory. I've never had a moment's regret; not one.

In years gone by, doctors refused to sterilize a woman unless she obeyed the '120 rule'. In other words, her age, multiplied by the number of children she had, must add up to at least 120. This rule has more or less disappeared now, but you will still encounter opposition if you are young and have never had children. The same goes for men. And the reluctance is probably a good thing, since it helps to prevent too many people from making mistakes which they can never rectify.

Of course, sterilization is not the answer for everyone. Some men and women feel 'unsexed' by the operation. And if the idea of being sterilized fills you with terror, don't even consider it.

Epilogue

The decision for or against having children is the most important one you will ever make. It will affect not only yourselves, but also any children you may one day have. The aim of this book has been to help you and your partner arrive at a decision which best reflects your own needs, desires and capabilities; and which takes account of the limiting factors which influence all our actions.

The decision-making process can be an arduous one, and it may be that you are unsure about whether or not you are 'parent material'. If so, counselling and co-counselling can help you to work through any unresolved conflicts (and some useful addresses are given at the end of the book).

Whatever choice you make, there are bound to be times when you find yourselves wondering what it would have been like had you chosen differently. For every choice there is a loss; for every decision, a denial. But there are tremendous benefits, too, in making a positive, conscious decision. Parenthood is too important a job to be allowed just to 'happen'.

Further Reading

So you want to have a baby? Tony Bradman (Julia MacRae 1985)
Test-tube Women R. Arditti et al. (Pandora Press 1984)
The Gift of a Child Elizabeth and Robert Snowden (Allen & Unwin 1984)
Coping with Childlessness Diane and Peter Houghton (Allen & Unwin 1984)
A Child by Any Means Maggie Jones (Piatkus Books 1989)
The Myth of Motherhood Elizabeth Badinter (Souvenir Press 1982)
Mad to be a Mother Brigid McConville (Century 1987)
Be Assertive Beverley Hare (Macdonald Optima 1988)
Relate guides to relationships and sexuality

| *Useful Addresses*

General organizations for people without children

British Organization of Non-Parents (BON)
BM Box 5866
London WC1N 3XX

Publishes a regular newsletter

ISSUE National Fertility Association (formerly National Association of Childless Couples)
318 Summer Lane
Birmingham B19 3RL
Tel. 021–359 4887
Helpline 021–359 7359

£30 to join, £15 to renew membership

Counselling and guidance

British Infertility Counselling Association
c/o BUPA Hospital Norwich
Old Watton Road
Colney
Norwich NR4 7TD

Association of those involved as counselling professionals

British Association for Counselling
37a Sheep Street
Rugby CV21 3BX
Tel. 0788–78328

Co-counselling
Send SAE for directory to:
Co-counselling Phoenix
Change Strategies
5 Victoria Road
Sheffield S10 2DJ

Relate (formerly Marriage Guidance)
Listed locally in telephone directories

Head Office:
Herbert Gray College
Little Church Street
Rugby CV21 3AP
Tel. 0788–573241

Association for Marriage Enrichment
c/o Westminster Pastoral Foundation
23 Kensington Square
London W8 5HN

Assertiveness

Redwood Women's Training Association
Invergarry
Kitlings Lane
Walton-on-the-Hill
Stafford ST17 0LE

Send £1 for programme of classes. This organization is country-wide, and offers classes for both men and women.

Your local college or adult education centre will probably also have details of assertiveness and self-awareness courses.

Adoption

British Agencies for Adoption and Fostering (BAAF)/Be My Parent
11 Southwark Street
London SE1 1RQ
Tel. 071–407 9763

£5 annual subscription

PPIAS (Parent to Parent Information on Adoption Services)
Lower Boddington
Daventry
Northants NN11 6YB

Advice and support for prospective adopters

National Foster Care Association (NFCA)
Francis House
Francis Street

London SW1P 1DE
Tel. 071-828 6266
£21.50 annual subscription

Post Adoption Centre
8 Torriano Mews
Torriano Avenue
London NW5 2RZ
Tel. 071-284 0555

LAGFAN (Lesbian and Gay Fostering and Adoption Network)
c/o London Friends Ltd
86 Caledonian Road
London N1 9DN
Holds regular monthly meetings and offers advice and support

Fertility investigations, pregnancy, sterilizations

BPAS (British Pregnancy Advisory Service)
First Floor
Guildhall Buildings
Navigation Street
Birmingham B2 4BT
Tel. 021-643 1461
Or check Yellow Pages for details of your nearest clinic

Lesbian and gay parenting

LAGFAN
c/o London Friends Ltd
86 Caledonian Road
London N1 9DN

Rights of Women
52/54 Featherstone Street
London EC1Y 8RT
Tel. 071-251 6577

Help and advice for parents

CRY-SIS
Tel. 071–404 5011

Parents Anonymous
8 Manor Gardens
London N7 6LA
Tel. 071–263 8918

Stillbirth and Neonatal Death Society (SANDS)
28 Portland Place
London W1N 4DE
Tel. 071–436 7940

Single parents

Gingerbread
35 Wellington Street
London WC2E 7BN
Tel. 071–240 0953

National Council for One Parent Families
255 Kentish Town Road
London NW5 2LX
Tel. 071–267 1361

Child and family welfare

NSPCC
67 Saffron Hill
London EC1N 8RS
Tel. 071–242 1626

Genetic disorders

Genetic Interest Group (GIG)
c/o Institute of Molecular Medicine
John Radcliffe Hospital
Headington

Oxford
OX3 9DU

An organization bringing together over fifty organizations and groups concerned with genetic disorders. GIG has a helpline, to give contact with individual support groups.

Index

absentee mothers 16
adoption 70–83; age limits for 72; overseas 71–2; process of 72–4; pros and cons of 86–7; qualifications for 72, 74–6
alternatives to childbearing 70–87
approval, need for 15–16
Association for Marriage Enrichment (AME) 101–4
attitudes to non-parents 9–12, 20, 88–95; coping with 88–95

BAAF 73, 82
'Be My Parent' 73
birth defects 40–1
British Association for Counselling 101
British Organisation of Non-Parents (BON) 42–7, 57, 61–9

childfree living 20–1, 41–7, 96–108
childlessness 10–11, 14, 28–35, 96–7
Childlink 77
children: reasons for wanting 13–27
Children's Society 75
conflict 58–61, 100–4; resolving 100–4
counselling 100–4; British Association for 101

'decidophobia' 57–8
decision-making 57–69
Down's Syndrome 40

environmental considerations 7

family pressures 13–16
fatherhood 4, 22–4
fertility: problems with 28–35; screening for 33–4
financial effects of parenthood 47–8
fostering 82–3
friendships 13–14, 17, 104–5

genetic counselling 39
GIFT 29
government: attitudes and policy 4–7
Green movement 7, 51–2

hereditary disorders 38–40

infertility 10–11, 14, 28–35; emotional impact of 31–2; fears of 26–7; male 4; treatments for 28–35;
ISSUE 30, 33
IVF 7, 28, 29, 30, 32, 34

LAGFAN 85–6
late motherhood 7
lesbian relationships 17
lesbian and gay adoption 75
lesbian and gay fostering 84–6

lesbian and gay parenting 83–6
Lewisham Home Finders 75
London Marriage Guidance 15

Madonna *see* Virgin Mary
Marriage Enrichment 101–4
material instinct 16–21
media 7–9
motherhood: and incidence of clinical depression 18; and desire for control 18–21; images of 16; in other countries 3–7; late 7, 26; myths and 2–4

NFCA 83
'New Man' 8–9, 24
non-parents: attitudes to 9–12, 20
NSPCC 67–8

parenthood: conflict and 58–61; decision-making 58–69; financial cost of 47–8; hereditary disorders and 38–40; ideological considerations 51–2; illness, disability and 36–8; lifestyle and 48–50, 63–5; mental illness and 39–40; motivation for 13–27, 65–6; relationships, effects on 13, 21–7, 48–50; second families 53–6; single 52–3

PPIAS 80
pressures to have children 13–27

Relate 101
relationships 13–14, 17, 48–50, 99–105

second families 53–6
self-assertion 94–5
single parenthood 52–3
society: and non-parents 11–12; pressures of 13–16, 42–3
sterilization 106–7

Virgin Mary, ideal of 2, 3, 11

Women's Movement 7–8